the
sustainable
diet

Includes over 100 delicious recipes
that are good for you AND the planet

SCOTT GOODING

First published in Australia and New Zealand in 2019 by Hachette Australia Pty Ltd

First Published in Great Britain in 2019
by Headline Home
an imprint of Headline Publishing Group

First published in paperback in Great Britain in 2022
by HEADLINE HOME
an imprint of HEADLINE PUBLISHING GROUP

1

Cataloguing in Publication Data is available from the British Library

ISBN 978 1 4722 9036 6
e-ISBN 978 1 4722 7359 8

MIX
Paper from
responsible sources
FSC® C104740

Headline's policy is to use papers that are natural, renewable and recyclable products and made from wood grown in sustainable forests. The logging and manufacturing processes are expected to conform to the environmental regulations of the country of origin.

Text design by Bookhouse, Sydney
Typeset in 12/16.3 pt Adobe Caslon Pro by Bookhouse, Sydney
Printed and bound in Great Britain by Clays Ltd, Elcograf S.p.A.

HEADLINE PUBLISHING GROUP
An Hachette UK Company
Carmelite House
50 Victoria Embankment
London EC4Y 0DZ

www.headline.co.uk
www.hachette.co.uk

To three people in particular: my two boys, Tashi and Zan, and you, *the reader.*

I would love for my boys to grow up with a different food landscape than what we currently have, with greater thought, consideration and emphasis on food sovereignty – for the betterment of human health, the health of the environment and animal welfare. For that to happen, it all comes down to us!
I hope that you read something in this book and implement it in your own world, sparking a deviation from the status quo. In order for large-scale change to happen or a shift in attitude to occur, it must begin with the individual. Collectively we can create a ripple of positive change. We all have a voice, one which can move us forward as a household, a village, a city, a country and a planet.

Contents

Foreword   ix
Introduction   xiii

PART ONE **UNDERSTANDING SUSTAINABILITY**

My top ten strategies for success   5
ONE   From foraging to factory farming   9
TWO   Is eating animal products good for us . . . and the
         environment?   29
THREE   Is veganism the answer?   47
FOUR   Is keto sustainable for you and the planet?   67
FIVE   Daily rhythms   83
SIX   Investing in your health   101
SEVEN   Conclusion   123

PART TWO **RECIPES FOR A SUSTAINABLE DIET**

Introduction to recipes   129
Breakfast   131
Lunch   147
Dinner   185
Sides   223
Sauces, dips and drinks   237

Endnotes   262
Further reading   265
Acknowledgements   266
Index   267

Foreword

I've got three superheroes. I'm in the entertainment business, so you might be surprised by who they are – they're definitely not the usual caped crusaders. Not film-makers nor artists, not community leaders, feminists or even public intellectuals, but farmers. Yes, farmers. A new breed of farmer: restorative farmers like Joel Salatin, Allan Savory and Isabella Tree. There are many more of their ilk, but these three have left their mark on me. They have renewed my hopes of combating climate change and changed how I want to farm and how I want to eat.

I have a small cattle farm on the North coast of Sydney and in recent years I have become increasingly interested in the ethics and environmental considerations of raising cattle. Animal welfare is important to me. Then there is the production of methane and the use of fertiliser and pesticides, which are real challenges for the farmer considering their role in climate change. How long could I ignore my personal responsibility? I knew my own cattle were well cared for, but what were they contributing to methane gas production and, more importantly, how was I degrading the land or polluting the river. I was contemplating returning my farmland to wilderness or swapping out cattle for the less impactful production of blue-berries or macadamia trees when the notion of 'regenerative farming' started to filter through the aether. Miraculously and unbeknownst to me, my farm manager, Mick, was already researching the very same notion.

It's been three years since Mick implemented the practices preached by my heroes on our farm. We now apply a natural cycle of herd concentration and movement and use natural waste fertilisers. We leave less-palatable grasses to the birds, rodents and insects. We have reduced our use of chemical drenches for internal and external parasites. We have ceased use of virtually all herbicides. Our transition from the old way to regenerative ways of farming is ongoing. Our goal is still to produce meat for profit, but with a focus on sustainability, particularly of long-term soil health.

Commensurately, more and more consumers want to know that the food they are buying is not only delicious and nutritious but is produced with consideration for the environment and animal welfare. Meals inspired by the endless stream of cookbooks on the market and television cooking shows may look delicious and help to impress dinner guests, but they pay scant attention to provenance of food and will do nothing for health outcomes and the Western epidemic of heart disease and obesity.

Enter Scott Gooding. As both health guru and chef, Scott recognises not only that these topics are in the zeitgeist but understands that health outcomes are irrevocably entwined with food provenance. With *The Sustainable Diet*, Scott has drawn together the disparate threads of growing right and eating right and shown us that there is an optimally healthy and ethical way forward.

I was a Scott convert after I was diagnosed with very high cholesterol. A doctor recommended that I begin taking statins, but Scott gave me advice on changing my diet. Dropping gluten, sugars and dairy did the trick very quickly. My cholesterol is now normal without medication and, even better, I discovered that I lost none of the enjoyment of my meals without the naughty bits. Scott has a knack for replacing the ingredients you thought you could never do without with something just as flavoursome or with a surprisingly fresh twist.

With this book, Scott may join my list of superheroes. I'm not sure I'm a convert to his insect recipes but I am sure my copy of *The Sustainable Diet* is not for loan.

Rachel Ward

Introduction

Let's face some cold, hard facts right from the get-go. Never in the history of humankind has the world been so populated. Never have there been so many people living with disease. And never has the environment been so vulnerable to the actions and behaviours of human beings. We have allowed capitalism to run riot, and the result is poor health on a global scale – both human and ecological. No-one is benefiting, aside from those knee-deep in large agribusiness.

We've lost sight of our species' past, eating foods that would have been unrecognisable to our ancestors, produced in ways that would seem entirely alien to them. Ancient farming practices have been abandoned in favour of intensive modern methods that rely heavily on the use of pesticides and fertilisers. Humankind has become domesticated, much like our livestock – buying what the big food companies want us to. Fresh, wild, organic produce – our staple diet since we first evolved – has been crowded out by highly processed and nutrient-poor foods, all in the space of a hundred years. It's time to get in touch with our wild side and break free of this enforced domestication. It's time to question everything, literally from the ground up: what we grow and how we grow it, what we eat and how we eat it – even when we eat it!

Our modern agricultural and nutritional models are fundamentally flawed. We're theoretically able, using current systems, to feed the entire world, but the reality is that more than 820 million people don't have enough to eat.[1] That's about one in nine. Many more eat a diet deficient in nutrients. Inequality, ill-health and disease – nobody wants or deserves that. A future in which food is fresh and nourishing and everyone has enough to eat shouldn't be a utopian dream, but can we nourish the Earth while we nourish ourselves, caring for its health as we care for our own? The answer to this question is complex and requires a concerted global effort, not to mention a shift in attitudes, but there are some simple, practical and affordable choices we can make every day to sustain our health *and* that of the planet.

The Sustainable Diet starts by looking at the industrial farming methods we use today and explores the alternatives. I've included case studies of farmers who've been inspired to go back to old ways, managing the land and producing food using strategies that mimic nature. Next I look at meat, and whether it's good for us, and then I ask if veganism might be the answer to our problems. I personally eat meat and fish, but I don't subscribe to the factory-farmed food system, and I believe it's important to ask these sorts of questions regardless of your own dietary persuasion.

I won't spend much time on specific diets, though I do include a brief chapter on keto, exploring if it might be an option for you. I'm not just looking at what is sustainable for the Earth and for agriculture, but the food behaviours and broader health choices that are sustainable for you, whatever your circumstances. I'm not interested in short-term detoxes, quick fixes or crash weight loss – this book is about what we can all do to live a healthy life over the long term. As such, I also look at our daily rhythms – when we wake, eat, exercise and sleep – and how we can learn to work with them, not against them, for optimum wellbeing. Part one ends with advice about investing in your health, with tips for how to shop and improve your cooking game.

Part two is full of recipes I've developed using sustainably produced foods that will also sustain good health – recipes that entirely embrace whole and fresh food, helping to significantly move the needle towards long-term health. It's important to consider the health of the planet as well as individual human health when cooking, along with respecting animal welfare if you choose to eat animal products.

Sustainability, by its very nature, is not just a buzzword – it's about taking the long view. The positive steps we take towards this goal must be achievable time and time again – today, tomorrow and for the rest of our days. We have the power to feed ourselves ethically produced, nourishing foods, grown by farmers whose concern for the land and their stock is at the heart of everything they do – it's just a matter of commitment. And we have the power to establish, and stick to, routines that will ensure optimum health. I'm hoping *The Sustainable Diet* will be a conversation starter, because the questions I raise in this book affect not only you and me, but our children and future generations – not to mention the health of the planet and the welfare of millions of animals.

PART ONE

Understanding sustainability

My top ten strategies for success

- Eat whole, fresh and as much unprocessed food as possible
- Go gluten free
- Limit industrialised oils
- Exercise and play regularly
- Hero the veggies
- Make meat the condiment
- Trace your food to its source
- Be open-minded to change
- Make decisions for your future self and your kids
- Be your own health detective

My top ten strategies for success

What do I mean by 'sustainable' – and, for that matter, 'success'? Well, when I talk about 'sustainable' I mean our obligation to the environment and to ethical farming practices that result in nutrient-rich foods, but I'm also talking about establishing a set of habits that promote good health. 'Success' is simply about making those habits permanent. Below are my top ten strategies for doing the best by you *and* the environment.

EAT WHOLE, FRESH AND AS MUCH UNPROCESSED FOOD AS POSSIBLE

Eating a broad range of fresh and unprocessed foods ensures a diversity of the life-enhancing vitamins and minerals needed to optimise and sustain your health. Highly processed foods are nutrient poor and can be harmful to your wellbeing when consumed in moderate or high quantities.

GO GLUTEN FREE

A gluten-free diet can be beneficial, and not just for those with coeliac disease – and it is easier than ever to find gluten-free products at the supermarket. Gluten can stimulate the protein zonulin, which disrupts the integrity of the gut membrane; increased gut permeability can wreak havoc on your wellbeing. Avoiding or limiting gluten in your diet has been found to help gut health and keep inflammation at bay. Inflammation is part of the body's immune response to perceived threats, and systemic inflammation is often the cornerstone of ill-health and disease. A major contributor to inflammation is gluten found in wheat, barley or rye products.

LIMIT INDUSTRIALISED OILS

Highly processed and industrialised oils have only been part of human diets in the last century and can be harmful to your health. Cutting down on highly processed oils will limit inflammation caused by free radicals derived from omega-6 fatty acids found in oils such as sunflower, safflower, bran, canola and vegetable. Instead, when cooking or dressing your foods, use macadamia, walnut, coconut and olive oils, or tallow, lard, ghee or butter.

EXERCISE AND PLAY REGULARLY

Regular exercise has been shown to elevate your Brain Derived Neurotrophic Factor (BDNF), which many call fertiliser for the brain, helping to grow and repair neurones. As well as helping to lift mood and combat anxiety and depression, exercise can help with insulin sensitivity and muscle tone. The key to making exercise habitual and sustainable is to choose a modality that is enjoyable or social. Social exercise helps to form bonds and improves interpersonal connections.

HERO THE VEGGIES

Vegetables should be celebrated. When designing your meal, start with the vegetables as the key ingredient, and then decide on the protein. The more varied and diverse your plant intake, the more varied and diverse the micronutrients you consume. Veggies have a bad rap, but you can liven up any vegetable with some delicious oils or butter, and dressings such as lemon juice or sea salt. Ensure your veggie intake includes 2–3 servings of dark green, leafy veg; 2–3 servings of red, orange, blue or purple berries or veg; and 1–2 servings of sulphur-rich veggies, such as onions or broccoli.

MAKE MEAT THE CONDIMENT

Too often the meat is the hero of the plate, with the salad or vegetables as an afterthought. Try to flip that approach on its head and treat the protein as the condiment to the vegetables. For each meal, you should have 3 fist-sized servings of aboveground veggies, 1 palm-sized serving of protein and 1–2 tablespoons of healthy fats.

TRACE YOUR FOOD TO ITS SOURCE

Understanding where your food has come from is an important part of the sustainable diet approach. A little bit of research into a brand's ethos or story can unearth whether their values align with yours on the topics of the welfare of animals and the use of fertilisers and pesticides.

BE OPEN-MINDED TO CHANGE

The health landscape is an ever-evolving beast with new and interesting discoveries occurring all the time. Keep your ear to the pulse and be willing to change in the interest of your health.

MAKE DECISIONS FOR YOUR FUTURE SELF AND YOUR KIDS

The decisions and choices made today can have a big impact (negative or positive) on your future. You may not notice it today or next week, but poor food and lifestyle choices *will* bite you on the bum further down the track. Your health is largely determined by epigenetics, that is external factors rather than your inherited genes – I'll discuss this later in the book – but this means that your behaviour is key. You are in control of the food choices for yourself and for your family, so it is important to make considered, informed decisions.

BE YOUR OWN HEALTH DETECTIVE

Don't accept the status quo or settle for ordinary – we are all entitled to be strong and healthy. Become a health vigilante by asking questions, reading food labels and listening to current research on health and the environment. Ask your fishmonger, butcher or local café where their produce comes from. Talking to others about sustainable choices is a step in the process – we're all in this together.

Chapter one

From foraging to factory farming

Before we can understand how our food is produced today and try to imagine how that might change in the future, we have to understand how we fed ourselves in the past. We're going to start by going back in time . . . way back, to a time before farming began. Then I'll take a look at how farming developed and examine how the food we eat today is produced – and why it's just not sustainable into the future.

THE FIRST FARMERS

If you're thinking about skipping this first part, recalling dull history lessons at school, don't! The story of food is the story of the entire human race – the story of how we've survived, and how we can survive the challenges we're facing now – so sit tight and read on!

The first Homo sapiens were hunter–gatherers, and they roamed their own particular territories, which they knew intimately, in small bands. They followed the cycle of the seasons, timing their travels to the fruiting of wild plants and the movement of migrating animals. Hunting gets all the glory, but gathering was just as important: our ancestors caught and ate small mammals, reptiles and insects, and foraged for edible grasses, leaves, flowers, seeds, nuts, berries and roots. Then, about 10,000 years ago, some clever folks came up with the idea of 'taming' plants and growing them as crops right on their own doorstep, so they'd no longer need to forage for them.

In parts of the world where foraging gave way to farming, human society was changed irrevocably. Growing crops meant staying nearby, to tend them, and so the first small villages were established. As the nomadic lifestyle started to give way to a more sedentary one, the food we ate changed too. Since switching to agriculture, humans have relied on a small number of staple crops – such as wheat, rice, corn and beans – as the basis of our diet. The problem is that these staple foods lack the diversity of nutrients supplied by a rich and varied diet. Early farmers suffered from this lack of diversity in the foods they ate. The most dramatic evidence of this was a drop in height. Their skeletons show us that the average male farmer was about 10 centimetres shorter than his hunting-and-gathering forefathers, who stood around 1.7 metres tall. Farmers were also more prone to cavities and other dental problems than their nomadic ancestors.

Their new way of life made them more vulnerable to illness, too. Staple crops could be harvested in greater quantities than their wild counterparts and stored to guard against seasonal shortages, which meant they could support bigger communities. As small villages grew into larger villages and eventually into towns, where thousands of people lived in close proximity for the first time, the risk of infectious disease grew. Over time, these early farmers also domesticated animals, including cows, sheep, goats, pigs and poultry, so they'd have a reliable supply of meat, milk and eggs – but living with animals at close quarters also exposed humans to new diseases they hadn't encountered before. Another problem, of course, was that crops were vulnerable to disease and drought. Hunter–gatherers could move on in the lean times, seeking more bountiful food in other parts of their territory – but once you've built a house, cleared fields and become integral to the community, you're not so keen to up sticks.

THE FAMILY FARM

Fast forward to the turn of the twentieth century and we find agriculture had fixed its roots steadfastly into society, entirely eclipsing hunter–gathering in the first world. Farming for crops and domesticating animals was a much more efficient and reliable method of food collection. Over time small holdings were established, allowing families to become self-sufficient while having the potential to earn money or produce tradable commodities. A small holding is an area of land that can be dedicated to growing several types of crops and housing pigs, horses, geese or cattle – smaller than a farm, but larger in scale than a few veggie plants in your backyard. During this time, the typical American farmer was able to feed six to eight people. Today the average American farmer feeds 126 people.

Small holdings or family farms failed to deliver the diverse nutrients that the hunter–gatherers experienced thousands of years prior. Despite the lowered nutrient diversity, this period of agriculture still produced organic, pesticide/fertiliser-free crops, from mineral-rich soils, which is an improvement on today's farming.

THE CONTEMPORARY FOOD INDUSTRY

Contemporary farming relies on 'monocropping', that is, growing a single crop on one piece of land for year after year – and it is now done on such a massive scale that a single species, such as corn or wheat, can occupy fields for kilometres at a stretch. Farmers have adopted this strategy in response to demand: they are not just feeding growing human populations but also supplying feed for livestock. This approach has obvious advantages for the farmer: it's much simpler to supply the needs of a single type of plant, and it makes crops easier to harvest, too, because it can be done with automated machinery. Monocultures don't exist in nature, though, and there's a reason for that.

Diverse ecosystems are kept in balance naturally by the mammals, birds and insects they are home to. When land is cleared for the planting of crops, many animals are driven from their former habitat, and that natural balance is upset. A particular species of insect might thrive in the new environment, for example, because it now has plentiful food. Just imagine the excitement of a hungry insect when confronted with vast swathes of its favourite plant to eat! If the predators that kept its numbers in check are now gone, there's nothing to stop such a species from overpopulating until it reaches plague proportions. A swarm of insects can devastate an entire crop in a matter of hours, and then move on to the next farm . . . and the next . . .

Another problem is that monocropping affects soil health. When the same stretch of land is repeatedly planted and harvested, the soil is depleted of nutrients. The result is less resilient plants, more vulnerable to disease – and to those voracious pests we've just been talking about. Having eliminated the natural checks and balances that a diverse ecosystem provides, monocropping farmers have to find ways to replicate them, at the same time doing whatever they can to support the overworked soil – which brings us to the subject of pesticides and fertilisers.

Pesticides

Intensive agribusiness doesn't work *with* nature but rather attempts to control, manipulate and manage nature. In a bid to maximise crop yields and increase profitability, nothing is left to chance – and the use of pesticides on crops is a prime example of this. Since the mid-twentieth century, there has been widespread use of pesticides to mitigate the damage done to crops by insects, weeds and rodents. The very first pesticides used highly toxic chemicals such as arsenic and hydrogen cyanide, but these were abandoned as they were too harmful or ineffective, paving the way for new pesticides to be synthesised.

The upside of using pesticides is higher yields – but the downside is that they don't just kill species that threaten crops, they're toxic to other species, too, including humans. DDT was heralded as the best thing since sliced bread: a pesticide that was effective and cheap to manufacture. But it was revealed to be incredibly detrimental to other creatures in the food chain, including fish and birds who were exposed. New generations of pesticides are water soluble and designed to contaminate less soil as they protect the crops, but they are no less toxic.

People who work with agricultural pesticides are most at risk from inhalation or exposure through skin contact, but the rest of us are more likely to ingest small traces in the food we eat. Residues can be found in a variety of everyday foods and drink, and washing and peeling fruits and vegetables isn't a bulletproof solution. The effect on our health will depend on the type and quantity of the pesticide, how we were exposed to it, and for how long. Our general health before exposure plays a part too. In some cases our bodies metabolise and excrete these toxic substances; in others, the pesticides accumulate in our body fat. Some pesticide residues have even been found in breastmilk samples.[1] Exposure has been linked to numerous illnesses, including cancer and a whole host of dermatological, gastrointestinal, neurological, respiratory, reproductive and endocrine disorders.[2]

If it were just toxic pesticides that farmers were using, it would be bad enough – but they also rely heavily on fertilisers to give their growing plants a leg-up.

Fertilisers

Soil quality and fertility has been the preoccupation of farmers for thousands of years. Egyptians and early Europeans would add manure to the soil to improve its mineral density. Nitrogen and phosphorus are essential to all living things, but intensive farming has depleted their presence in the soil. As a result, large-scale industrial agriculture has come to rely on commercially produced fertilisers containing these nutrients. More often than not, the mentality when applying fertilisers has been 'the more, the better'. After rain, the excess runs off and contaminates neighbouring waterways. High levels of nutrients in the water may lead to toxic algal blooms, causing oxygen levels to drop. Those plants living there and the animals that can't get away fast enough end up dying off, and these rivers that should be abundant with life become 'dead zones'.

The Gulf of Mexico, which should be teeming with life, is now a dead zone, as tributaries pass through agricultural land before reaching the ocean. The zone occurs between the inner and mid-continental shelf in the northern Gulf of Mexico, beginning at the Mississippi River delta and extending westward to the upper

Texas coast, covering an area of up to 10,000 square kilometres. Because fish and other commercial species usually move out to sea in order to avoid the dead zone, fishermen are forced to travel farther from land – and spend more time and money – to make their catches, adding stress to an industry already hurt by hurricanes and the oil spill.

Similarly, intensive agriculture in the Great Barrier Reef catchment has resulted in substantial nutrient input into coastal waters. I first visited the Great Barrier Reef in 1999 and was lucky enough to dive just off Green Island – even back then the effects of global warming (coral bleaching) and fertiliser run-off was evident. The Great Barrier Reef was once an ecological nirvana – sadly this no longer is the case. Since 2003, the Australian and Queensland governments have implemented a range of initiatives to fight the pollution of the reef, including a monitoring program that measures water quality entering the reef's lagoon. An estimated 12,000 tonnes of nitrogen and 2900 tonnes of phosphorus came from monitored catchments in 2014–15.[3] But despite these efforts, total nitrogen entering the Great Barrier Reef is still rising, and it's doubtful that current strategies will be enough to reach the targets that the government initiatives are aiming for.[4]

These sorts of man-made environmental disasters are being addressed through tighter regulation of the use of fertilisers. The challenge is to use an adequate amount of fertiliser to support crops as they grow without harming the environment. But limiting our use of fertilisers isn't enough. If nothing is done to remedy the current situation, then we'll soon need to use even more fertiliser to counteract the further degradation of the soil, or clear new land for farming . . . and neither option is a positive solution, nor sustainable.

THE WESTERN DIET

At the start of this book, I said that the number of people on this planet living with disease is unprecedented. Think about that for a second. We have sophisticated methods of farming, and rapid forms of refrigeration, transportation and distribution. We also have incredible methods of diagnosis, state-of-the-art hospitals and medical technology, and highly trained and expert health professionals. And yet, despite all that, the number-one cause of mortality in wealthy countries like Australia and the UK is non-communicable diseases – many of which are caused by poor diet and lifestyle choices.

The Western lifestyle, complete with intensive food systems, has systemically ravaged human and ecological health. The industrialised world has fallen victim to being undernourished while simultaneously being overfed. It sounds like an oxymoron, but the average Western diet is deplete in the necessary minerals and nutrients to allow us to thrive. The global staple foods in the industrialised world are corn, sugar, wheat, rice, soy, maize, and ground beef from feedlot livestocks – it's a recipe for poor health. These commodities are shoulder-charging fresh, nutrient-rich produce out of the way.

We are bombarded daily with nutrient-poor food choices. It's no coincidence that processed and packaged foods use cheap commodities such as grains, sugar and corn to keep the price point low and lure the consumer in. The combination of sweet, salt and fat is no coincidence either, these foods hit all our pleasure points in a way that nothing in nature does.

We are witnessing unprecedented numbers of obesity, diabetes and heart disease both domestically and internationally. An estimated 1 million Australian adults (5 per cent) had type 2 diabetes in

2014–15, according to self-reported data from the ABS 2014–15 National Health Survey.[5] There were 16,400 Australian deaths in 2015 due to diabetes, with half of these (55 per cent) due to type 2 diabetes. In the UK, one in ten people over forty are living with type 2 diabetes, according to Diabetes UK. The status quo simply isn't serving any of us well.

USING NATURE AS A TEMPLATE

We have lost the connection to the earth with our modern farming practices – there's simply no room for it in intensive farming. The need to maximise profits erases any consideration of animal welfare or the health of the land. Large-scale farm operators work in opposition to nature rather than capitalising on nature's drive to grow, support, bind and flourish.

Nature has a curious way of surviving. Plants will support and protect one another, creating pathogen barriers collectively and warning one another against predation. Their ability to communicate largely occurs through the mycelium, a complex and sophisticated network of tendrils, roots and neurotransmitters – somewhat like a subterranean internet. Mycelia are essentially the roots' system for fungi, but one which all plants can communicate through. It's worth noting that the largest living organism on the planet is a mycelium in a forest in Oregon (not the Great Barrier Reef, as was commonly thought). It's also worth noting that 25 per cent of the Earth's biomass (that is, all living things) is of the fungi family.

American biologist E.O. Wilson states that the richness and diversity of life is dependent on a complex web of natural resources and species. The greater the biomass, the greater the productivity of the land and its resilience.[6] Sadly, the contemporary attitude to farming and subsequent misuse of land has resulted in a dramatic loss of biomass. In 2013 the State of Nature report compiled by British scientists from 25 wildlife organisations detailed how many species were in drastic decline worldwide: 60 per cent of species have declined in recent decades and one in ten species are at risk of disappearing altogether.[7]

If you've ever walked through a wild forest, it's blindingly evident that no species of plant grows either en masse or in isolation from other plants (like we see with intensive arable farming). Rather, there is rich diversity among living things. Nature naturally fosters a robust and complex microbe diversity, ensuring the soil is teeming with life. Crops grown intensively or hydroponically do not have exposure to microbes – and this has implications for our health. The microbes, pathogens, viruses, bacteria and yeast in our guts play a significant role in determining our state of health. A rich and diverse population is vital to good health.

On a side note, many studies have been undertaken with indigenous hunter–gatherers in Tanzania, specifically the Hadza tribes. It's been shown that their microbiome (once known as gut flora) is among some of the most diverse on the planet. Why is that? It's because their rich and varied diet, including zebra, lizards and insects, exposes them to microbes found in the earth, on animals and in nature, providing them with ideal gut health. Their food is *always* organic, biodynamic and free of harmful pesticides and fertilisers.

So my point is, rather than working against nature, as is evident with intensive farming, perhaps it is more beneficial to work *with* nature. Given that nature (when left alone) will strive for growth and biodiversity, perhaps we can develop food systems that help the earth and ensure the foods grown are richer in nutrients? The most successful farming practices will be ones that utilise nature rather than fight it head on. They will have no need to employ extreme contingency plans – as seen with pesticides and fertilisers.

'MOVING, MOBBING AND MOWING'

I'd like to introduce you to an American farmer by the name of Joel Salatin. In 1961, Joel and his father bought land in the Shenandoah Valley in Virginia. Historically, this valley had been incredibly fertile, providing the Native Americans who farmed it with ample sustenance for hundreds of years. Early European settlers ploughed the valley and planted it with grains, and it became the region's breadbasket. Over the course of the next 150 years, up to two and a half metres of topsoil was washed away and when Joel and his father went to install fences on the property, there wasn't enough soil to drive the posts into. What was once fertile land was now unworkable.

Joel and his father took a step back and observed how natural systems functioned, from the constant movement of animals across the land, to the cycle of building up and decomposing organic material. They pondered whether they might draw on nature as their ally.

First they dumped surplus corncobs (and any other organic matter they could source) on rock piles to help cultivate biomass, that is, more organic material. They placed fallen trees into gullies, with the butts facing downhill to slow the flow of water and diminish the harmful effects of fast-flowing water over land. Rocks were placed in the bottom of gullies to provide a dam for the water, slowing the water down even further and allowing for silt to be deposited uphill, forming terraces. The property included a forest. This provided an incubation zone for the biomass shortage in open land. They also invested in a wood chipper, allowing them to put more and more organic matter onto the land from the forest.

Over time, the biomass diversity improved, soil quality returned and the land became workable again.

Joel made another helpful observation, and that was that nature tends to favour perennials over annuals. Annuals, like corn and wheat, are plants that grow and make a seed, which needs replanting, in contrast to perennials which simply regrow, like many grasses and herbs.

Fast-cycling perennials are plants that sprout, grow and die quickly. If these plants are to continue to metabolise solar energy and stay green, they need to be pruned before they reach the end of their life cycle and die. This is achieved in nature by herbivores that graze the fast-cycling perennials, helping to maintain vegetation on the land. Joel created a protocol, which he termed 'Moving, Mobbing and Mowing', and replicated this on his farm. It was built upon the observation that herbivores, when left to their own devices, will naturally prune the fast-cycling perennials, fertilise the grazing area with manure and aerate the topsoil.

When we remove a herbivore from its natural occupation, the symbiotic relationship between plant/land and animal is interrupted and disharmony follows. Industrial farming, using herbivores, does not prescribe to the 'Moving, Mobbing and Mowing' mentality – instead it creates feedlots, in which cattle are penned and fed an unnatural diet of grains to manage their weight ahead of market and slaughter. Feedlots do not support the land or create healthy and happy cows, and ultimately they decrease the quality of the meat being farmed. It's mostly this meat that is consumed by humans on our planet.

Nearly 60 years after Joel's father first bought the property, the land is continuing to thrive and delivering fresh, organic produce. To this day, Joel farms pigs, chickens, turkeys, rabbits and vegetables supplying locals, restauranteurs and markets. Joel is a huge proponent of sustainable farming and working with nature to optimise the health of the land.

CELL GRAZING AND UNTOUCHED BORDERS

I'd like to bring things a little closer to home and introduce you to Mick Green, the farmer. Mick has been living on a property in Utungun, six hours drive from Sydney and 10 kilometres west of Macksville, New South Wales, since 2010. His father tended to the land before him since 1996. He is a loveable character and is incredibly passionate about regenerative farming. Much like Joel, Mick believes that mimicking nature on the farm benefits us all – humans, animals and plants – and the land too.

One way in which he mimics nature is through a strategy called 'cell grazing'. Livestock are rotated through a series of paddocks, or 'cells'. By the time they're done grazing the last paddock, the pasture in the first paddock has recovered, and the rotation can start again. The rest period is determined according to the plants' growth cycle, which helps to preserve the soil and protect the land.[8]

Cattle in their natural environment will mob together as a defence mechanism against predators. The mob ensures that all grasses in that cell (not just the sweet ones) are kept pruned and in a vegetative stage. This stage is when grasses are photosynthesising, and it helps to sequester carbon into the ground, as the growing blade of grass acts like a solar panel, taking in sunlight as well as carbon from the atmosphere and locking it into the earth. Cell grazing helps to ensure that a greater diversity of grasses are eaten before the cattle are moved on to a new cell of fresh grass – in Mick's case, every 24 hours.

Another way in which Mick works with nature is by leaving his borders untouched. The property that Mick works includes a number of dams. These are imperative to survival on Australian farms, as dry seasons can be very long in certain areas. Dams are water catchment areas over impermeable bedrock or clay. They can be natural or man-made. The dam creates a fringe or border with the open land, and on Mick's farm this junction is deliberately left a little 'wild' to create habitats for nesting creatures, including rodents and birds, ensuring biomass diversity on the property. The same rules are applied to fence lines or steep land, where vegetation is allowed to grow wild to help encourage a variety of animal species to lodge there, which all contribute to the overall biomass and health of the land.

Adherents of intensive farming have always said in defence of their practices that the world simply cannot be fed using a sustainable agricultural system. I asked Mick if he thought the planet could be fed using regenerative or sustainable food systems. I anticipated that he'd acknowledge that his approach was great for the land but that sadly it couldn't realistically feed 7-million-plus mouths. Well, you can imagine my pleasure when Mick replied, 'Shit yeah!'

There have always been organic farmers and regenerative advocates operating on the fringes, while the capitalist juggernauts of food production dominate the industry, but increased interest and investment from consumers and greater availability of organic and ethically sourced produce is on the up – a telling marker that maybe the pendulum is swinging back.

Rewilding

Isabella Tree performed a radical transformation on her prop-erty in Sussex in the United Kingdom.[9] The land had been intensively farmed for decades, resulting in degraded soil. She tried new machines and chemical products to yield more productivity from the land, but the farm couldn't be turned around. So Isabella and her husband decided to do something fairly unconventional. They allowed their land to 'rewild' – with no human intervention, they let the land regenerate itself and nature to take over.

They knew that each animal had a role to play, in how they walked the Earth, what parts of the plants they ate, the manure they produced. Although many of the species native to their part of the countryside were long gone, Isabella introduced species that best resembled them and sat back to let nature do its thing. She removed fences and drains. The end result was a thriving, enriched plot of land which, although it looked nothing like the farm they knew, was once again profitable.

Her story is echoed time and time again by regenerative farmers and conservationists – all of whom are advocates for working with the land rather than against it. It's a comforting story to hear, but we aren't out of the woods yet . . . still most of the farmed land in industrialised countries is done so intensively. The bottom line is that not all farming is done the same way, and one food system can look unrecognisable from another. We need to learn which ones to support as much as we can, for the sake of the environment and our health.

THE BENEFITS OF LIVESTOCK

I remember studying for my A-levels back in 1995 and answering an exam question on desertification – its causes and its impact on global warming. Everything I'd heard or read to that point indicated that grazing herds, particularly goats, cows and sheep, were a major contributor to desertification across vast areas of the globe. Not only were these grazing animals damaging the soil, but their methane output was incredibly detrimental to climate change.

Intensive farming clears the land, leaving the topsoil exposed to the elements and increasing fragility, and if monocrops are then planted, which perennially extract nutrients and minerals from the soil, driving farmers to add more and more fertilisers, the quality of soil declines over time. Damaged and exposed soils release carbon into the atmosphere, instead of staying in the dirt and vegetation (as nature intended). Carbons which are taken underground as part of this natural system are locked in the earth for hundreds if not thousands of years. This devastating desertification had rendered areas of the globe inhospitable to civilisation, relinquishing the opportunity for that land to be a source of food for the population.

That was certainly the message eighteen-year-old Scott (sporting my ponytail and baggy jeans) had received. I blithely agreed that livestock caused land degradation and global warming. It was only later that I came to believe that livestock could actually be part of the solution to *reversing* desertification.

Allan Savory is a Zimbabwean ecologist, livestock farmer, environmentalist, and president and co-founder of the Savory Institute, which runs education and conservation programs to promote large-scale restoration of the world's grasslands. Mr Savory believes that the only way to reverse desertification – and potentially climate change – is to use livestock animals to mimic nature – just as Joel Salatin, Isabella Tree and Farmer Mick have. In the wild, grazing herds form large packs in a bid to protect themselves from predation; the larger the group, the less risk each individual animal has to be attacked. A large herd will effectively urinate and poo (excuse my French) on its food, which encourages constant movement of the herd (because, let's face it, no-one wants poo on their food). It's this natural set of circumstances that encourages vegetation to proliferate. Vegetation helps to bind soil and ultimately reduce the carbon released into the atmosphere. The soil can also sequester the methane from the manure, given the right conditions. Mr Savory's findings strongly support the argument that, if managed the right way, livestock can help to reverse desertification . . . and might even, if managed the correct way on all the desertified areas of the globe, lower carbon in the Earth's atmosphere to pre-industrial levels.

Dom and the business of ethical produce

I first met Dom around ten years ago, when he was running a busy butcher's shop in the eastern suburbs of Sydney. The Grass Roots Urban Butchery – or GRUB, as it was called – was one of a kind, as far as I knew. Dom had opened his shop in response to his own desire for a one-stop shop for ethical produce. 'There was a want and need to find real food,' he explained to me, 'and going to the farmers' market every week was driving me nuts, so I said, "Let's do it ourselves."'

It wasn't long before word spread about what Dom was doing and the business grew. The next few years were a series of ups and downs. Dom's drive and passion for real food was somewhat thwarted by his inexperience as a trained butcher, and he learnt some hard lessons in business very quickly. During his stint at GRUB he met with an organic egg farmer. They soon formed a partnership and together went into egg production.

The land Dom bought needed a lot of help. Previous land-management strategies, which had included the use of pesticides, were stopped immediately. Dom took courses in regenerative farming and read as much as he could to ensure best practice.

Producing eggs sustainably comes with its own set of problems. His chickens are free range and organic and have access to pasture – which makes for happy chickens. However, chickens can be the victims of stress, just like us, which affects egg production. Where intensively farmed chickens are kept in climate-controlled sheds, lit to encourage feeding, and protected from predators, Dom's chickens had to survive with more limited safeguards. As a safety measure Dom has a perimeter fence, which is set deep into the ground to discourage foxes, as well as a mob of maremma dogs – an Italian sheepdog not to be messed with – which live inside the enclosures protecting the chickens.

Ethical and organic eggs are more expensive to produce, due to higher labour costs, higher feed costs and reduced bird density per hectare, compared to intensively farmed birds. Dom points out that this will always be the case with real, ethical produce. He echoes my position on our current food landscape, saying that we have placed value on the wrong sorts of food. 'We need to look at the way we shop, cook and eat,' he says. 'We have placed value on convenience foods and become so reliant on this that our health suffers, the environment suffers and it's confronting for people to see reason to pay extra for real, ethical produce. The need and desire comes when someone gets sick. Only at this point is the urge strong enough to engage in supporting the right food systems. Collectively we need to shop, cook and think smarter: don't eat so much, and look at the macronutrients. We don't need to be filling up on carbohydrates leaving us feeling hungry all the time but instead eating nutrient-dense good-quality food.' He adds, 'Feeling is believing. Most of us in the Western world don't know what it feels like to be healthy.'

Dom knows he's relatively new to the world of regenerative farming and admits that it has its challenges, but the reward is a feeling of integrity, and access to real food for his family. But isn't that what all of us want?

We have in our favour that humans are incredibly adaptive, responsive and possess such ingenuity that we have the ability to adopt new food systems . . . en masse! This, of course, won't happen globally overnight, it will take time to trickle down to the big agribusiness model, but sustainable farming practices are nothing radical or new – we just have to remind ourselves.

UNDERGROUND FARMING

The major difference between regenerative and intensive farming is the extent to which nature is mimicked or incorporated. Clearly, intensive farming attempts to overpower and control nature through interventions such as fertilisers, hormones, antibiotics and pesticides. There's nothing natural about giving blanket antibiotics to cattle, giving growth hormone to chickens or fertilisers to plants – but these measures optimise yields.

I'm not saying that controlling measures in farming can't be used in sustainable practices. It might sound like something from *Mad Max*, but underground farming is a growing industry when land on the surface is at a premium.

There is no weather 30 metres underground, so plants rely entirely on ingenious man-made systems. Underground farmers know how much light plants need to thrive, how much water and nutrients are required for their best growth. Water is delivered intermittently to mimic natural rain patterns, and carefully recycled. Energy-efficient timers control the temperature and CO_2 levels. The systems are steeped in science but are based on the natural model, with a sustainable backbone.

Key Takeaways

1. The current health guidelines and food systems are not serving human health or the health of the planet.
2. There are alternatives to intensive farming that can nourish the population while not proving detrimental to our ecosystem and the environment.
3. Have you ever questioned where your food comes from and which food system it was part of?

Chapter two

Is eating animal products good for us . . . and the environment?

Is eating meat good for us? People have been debating this for hundreds of years, and never more so than right now. With global epidemics of obesity, Alzheimer's and diabetes together with a threatened environment, people are looking for a solution, and it's meat and meat eaters in the crosshairs. The question of whether meat and seafood are sustainable food sources is contentious and controversial, but I'll attempt to ask exactly what we need to take into account to answer this as best I can. Eating meat and seafood is hinged on individual ethics, which is why it can be a loaded question, but I'll come to this later in the book.

LET'S TALK BEEF

To decide whether meat is good for us, we have to make a couple of assumptions. First, we have to assume that everyone is eating meat of the same quality. If this is our starting point, it's simply a matter of weighing up the nutritional pros and cons – but as I'm sure you'll have guessed, it's not that easy. Different approaches to farming produce meat of a different quality. Say one animal has been allowed to roam as it would in nature (or close to it), eating what it would in the wild, and the other has been kept in a pen, pumped full of antibiotics and fed an unnatural diet. As you'd imagine, the flesh of the first animal would be tastier – and more nutritious. For beef, these approaches are called 'grass-fed/-finished', where the livestock roam and feed in pasture until slaughter, and 'feedlot', where the cattle, once they reach a certain weight, are moved into pens and fed specialised animal feed designed for fast weight gain for the last six to eight months before slaughter.

The second assumption we have to make is that everyone is eating the same amount of meat – but we can't really assume that, either. Many of us who choose to eat meat arguably consume too much, whether grass-fed/-finished or otherwise. For the sake of the argument, though, I'd like to explore two scenarios. In both scenarios, we'll assume that the person in question is getting adequate protein. In the first, they'll be eating organic meat from a steer that has always been fed on grass, and in the second they'll be eating meat that was in a feedlot for up to a year before slaughter.

SCENARIO 1: grass-fed/-finished meat

Grass-fed/-finished meat has been shown to contain less overall fat, more beneficial fatty acids and more vitamins than feedlot beef. It's also a good source of a variety of nutrients. Compared to feedlot beef, grass-fed beef is higher in vitamins B_1 and B_2; vitamin E; betacarotene; calcium, magnesium and potassium.

The grass-fed beef's total omega-3s were higher too, as was its ratio of omega-3 to omega-6 fatty acids. These are essential fatty acids, but our bodies can't manufacture them, so we need to get them from our diet. It's the ratio of the two that we have to watch. Ideally the ratio of omega-3 to omega-6 should be around 1:2, but in the West it is heavily skewed in favour of omega-6, due to the industrialised oil and grains consumed, and can be as high as 15:1.[1] The omega profile of grass is far superior to that of feedlot staples such as grain and corn: as much as 60 per cent of the fatty acids found in grass are omega-3. Feedlot cattle can have two to four times the amount of omega-6 as their grass-fed counterparts.

Another point in favour of grass-fed/-finished meat is that it has fewer calories than that of feedlot animals, most likely due to its lower total fat content. Feedlot cattle are fed a high-carbohydrate diet to fatten them up ahead of slaughter. This, along with the animals' lack of mobility, makes it unsurprising that intensive farming methods produce fattier animals.

SCENARIO 2: feedlot-finished meat

Around 97–98 per cent of Australia's national beef herd, estimated at 24 million head, is located in pasture on extensive cattle properties, with the remainder within cattle feedlots. Despite the small number of cattle within feedlots, they contribute around 38 per cent of Australia's beef production.[2] This is because 'finishing' cattle on grain in a feedlot is quicker and more efficient than finishing them on grass. Cattle in feedlots are typically given growth hormones to promote weight-gain for market and slaughter. According to the Union of Concerned Scientists, up to six different growth hormones may be given to beef cattle in the US.

The same group of scientists also claim that a shocking 70 per cent of all antibiotics used in the US are fed to livestock.[3] Intensive farming crowds vast numbers of cattle in close proximity to each other, in less than sanitary conditions, thereby increasing the animals' exposure to pathogens, and to combat this, antibiotics are used. This is not to say that grass-fed/-finished cattle are immune to disease, but the conditions in which they live mean that the risk is reduced. Antibiotics also promote growth and farming efficiencies. In 2013, almost 15,000 tonnes of antimicrobials were sold and distributed for use in livestock.[4] This is a clear example of the extreme measures involved in farming against nature.

A window into a cow's stomach

Transfaunation – the act of taking microbes from one source and putting them in another – can help cows when they get sick. Designated donor cows with a surgically installed rumen fistula are kept in some veterinary colleges to allow access to the cow's rumen from the outside. A rumen fistula is a permanent hole between a cow's internal organs and the outside world. Essentially a fist-sized hole is created in the flank of the cow straight into the stomach, covered with a plastic casing. This gives instant access to the cow's rumen – a large part of their stomach responsible for digestion – to assess the health of its digestive system. A fistula can also allow us to understand how different nutrients and diets affect a cow's digestive system and can be pivotal to maximising the health of the farmer's assets and ultimately profit. Dr Susan Fubini, a professor of large animal surgery at Cornell University's College of Veterinary Medicine, says that the cow feels no pain and suffers no ill-effect from the procedure. Personally, I can't imagine the cow not experiencing any discomfort as a hole is created in its flank. Although it may be designed to benefit health, to me this radical, inhumane and bizarre practice that has become normalised by intensive farming, is another example of the fact that we have lost connection with the animals we farm and is reflective of how highly commoditised livestock has become. It sounds crazy to have a window into a cow's stomach, but that's the world we live in!

RUMINATING ON THE PROBLEM

Cows are ruminants – by nature they graze. Allowing cattle to graze on well-managed pastures from birth to slaughter is at the core of sustainable beef production. The animals raised in this way are often referred to as 100 per cent grass-fed. (From now on, when I say 'grass-fed', I mean 'grass-fed and finished'.) What's good for animal welfare is also good for the environment – and for consumers.

It has been suggested that, like for like, grass-fed cattle will produce more methane (a significant driver of climate change) than feedlot cattle. But it is also argued that grazing, when well-managed, can offset methane and other greenhouse gas production from cattle because vegetation soaks up and stores carbon, preventing carbon dioxide – another greenhouse gas – from being released into the atmosphere.

Grass-fed cattle require more acreage than feedlot cattle, but the environmental cost of intensively farmed livestock is greater. In order to feed cattle in feedlots, grains/soy/corn have to be grown and processed elsewhere, which means there are additional environmental costs, including, but not limited to, soil degradation, fertiliser run-off and pollution from transportation.

When animals are kept at appropriate stocking rates on well-managed grasslands or pasture, their manure is spread on the land at levels the pasture can handle. The nutrients can be returned to the soil and recycled – and actually improve the land instead of degrading it. This reiterates my earlier discussion on Joel Salatin and his 'Move, Mob, Mow' approach to managing cattle. (Incidentally, I reckon 'Move, Mob, Mow' has potential as a catchy pop song . . . I'll work on it.)

When comparing the health of grass-fed versus feedlot cattle, it's certainly worth pointing out that any animal (including us) will thrive best on a diet which is physiologically appropriate to them. I mentioned the Hadza tribe earlier, who have an organic hunter–gatherer diet, which results in an incredibly diverse gut microbiome – a strong indicator of health. Cattle that have access to green pastures grown on fertile soil, free of chemicals, have the greatest potential to be healthy.

As long as pasture is managed correctly, grass-fed cattle will be spared many of the diseases contracted by cattle reared in stressful and crowded conditions, and the need to administer antibiotics is reduced.

LAMB AND MUTTON

As beef is the meat most scrutinised for contributing to global warming, I have chosen to focus primarily on beef production, but it's certainly worth shining a light on the lamb industry. Australia is the world's largest exporter of sheep meat and the second largest exporter of mutton. Australia remains one of the only countries to export live sheep to foreign countries, which raises ethical questions around animal welfare. The sheep meat industry accounts for 36 per cent of all businesses within Australian agriculture.

As we have seen with cattle, there are different farming attitudes and practices which impact the welfare of an animal, the environment and human health, and lamb farming is no different. Until researching this book I was under the impression that sheep roamed the land at will and were truly free range, however that might not always be the case. Feedlots have become increasingly popular in the sheep industry, with sheep being intensively grain finished, to ensure the animal reaches the market specifications at the right time in order to maximise profits.

Two methods are used, one is feedlot within concrete stalls, limiting the animals' space to roam, quite similar to beef feedlots. The other is confined paddock feeding which is, as the name suggests, feeding grain from a man-made station in the open paddock. The confined paddock method can be useful in droughts, a hardship often experienced by Australian farmers.

In the UK, sheep tend to be pasture-raised and therefore grass-fed, but check the labels at the supermarket or ask your butcher.

PIGS

Pigs are not exempt from the disparities of farming methods. A pig either strikes it lucky and lands herself in a free-range farm or the confines of a stall inside a factory farm facility. The free-range pig will spend thirteen weeks with her mother, whereas the second pig will be weaned off her mother at ten days to maximise growth through controlled diets. The early removal from their mother's milk gives them a yearning to suck and chew, which is problematic for the curly tail of the pig in front, so many tails are clipped at birth.

Motherless and tailless pigs are confined to stalls with little to no exposure to sun, grass and wind. Conversely, free-range pigs are outdoors at all times with access to shelter for protection. For pork to be accredited free range, pigs need to be kept permanently outside from birth to death, with access to bedding material and shelter from the elements. Sadly only 5 per cent of pork in Australia is free range and even less is organic, usually from small farms. In the UK, free-range pork is becoming more widely available, but make sure you look for the free-range, organic or RSPCA-assured labels. Making conscientious choices around the pork you buy can contribute to the improvement of living conditions for pigs.

CHICKEN

A similar roll of the dice befalls the chicken too. One can either land herself in a crowded barn, pumped full of antibiotics and growth hormones, or luck out and land in a pasture-raised environment, free to scratch, head bob and peck all the insects, grubs and seeds she wants.

The conditions for chickens raised intensively are pretty grim. Thankfully the practice of caging hens, when the animal remained permanently in cages within a shed, is now taboo. I optimistically believe that in a relatively short period of time caged hens will be a grim but distant memory. However, we are not out of the woods yet – barn-raised hens is a step up but it still imposes on the health of the animal. Overcrowding in barns is a real issue for the hens' wellbeing, compounded by unnaturally accelerated growth causing instability and loss of movement – it's not a place a hen deserves to be. They also have to contend with unnatural hours of light, due to artificial lights inside the sheds, disrupting their circadian rhythm, along with issues such as cannibalism, toe removal, and nail and beak trimming.

That being said I feel the chicken and egg industry is changing and evolving quicker than any other meat industry. This, I believe, is largely down to a combination of ethical farmers, like Dom, and the consumer making informed decisions on which type of egg to support, thus putting pressure on big supermarkets.

NUTRITIONAL VALUES IN ANIMAL PRODUCTS

Even without taking ethics into consideration, there seems to be compelling evidence to favour grass-fed meat over intensive feedlot meat on the basis of nutrition. It is crucial to consider the quality of meat consumption as well as the quantity; in short, processed meats can be detrimental to your health.

Animal sources provide certain nutrients and minerals, such as vitamins B_{12} and D_3, taurine, creatine, heme iron and docosahexaenoic acid (DHA), of which some are unique to animal products. To choose to not eat meat could potentially lead to deficiencies – and to avoid the effects of those, supplementation is probably a wise idea.

Although it can be found in poultry and seafood, meat – especially red meat – is the best source of heme iron. Heme iron from meat is more bio-available – that is, easily absorbed by the body – than non-heme iron. An insufficient intake of iron may result in anaemia, which can result in weakness, dizziness, headaches, chronic fatigue or depression.

However, eating meat is not the only way to get iron in your diet. Non-heme iron is found in non-animal sources such as grains, rice and beans, and is also found in nuts, fruits, vegetables and seeds – but be aware that it is less bio-available and you may need to monitor your iron more closely if you are using these sources. There is a strong argument against eating copious amounts of meat. In *The Keto Diet* I dedicated an entire chapter to the idea that there's a tipping point when it comes to the health benefits of animal consumption, particularly if the end game is to achieve ketosis.

DHA is another interesting nutrient that you may not know. It is found in fatty fish (such as mackerel, sardines, salmon), and in lower concentrations in meat and eggs. It's also found in human breastmilk and is important for foetal brain development. My partner took DHA fish supplement consistently throughout her recent pregnancy. It's vital to maintenance of normal brain function in adults, too.[5] Supplementing with DHA is certainly worthwhile if your choice is to not eat meat, fish and eggs. Fortunately, DHA is commonly found in health food shops, chemists or online.

FARMED FISH VERSUS WILD FISH

The subject of farmed fish versus wild fish is a prickly one. Much as with the livestock food systems, it's not as easy as saying that natural is better. It actually comes down to good practice and ethical responsibility. There are good and bad fisheries within each sector.

'Wild-caught fish' evokes romantic images of man and his rod. It speaks to our DNA; it is something humans have done for thousands of years. Yet the reality of wild-caught fishing can be very unromantic and in fact quite horrifying. The global demand for fish has led to dragnet fishing and super trawlers. Some of these ships are capable of fishing continuously for weeks at a time. They can hold thousands of tonnes of fish and are indiscriminate about what gets caught in their nets.

At 144 metres long and weighing 14,055 tonnes, the *Annelies Ilena* is Europe's largest fishing vessel. This super trawler can hold 7000 tonnes of fish. Various other vessels of comparable size are at work the world over. The massive fishing capacity of these vessels have played a part in overfishing on a global scale, depleting stocks of Chilean jack mackerel in the South Pacific, as well as bigeye tuna and yellowfin tuna in the Coral Triangle, which includes the waters of Indonesia, Malaysia, Papua New Guinea and Solomon Islands. Additionally, there are the bycatch victims of indiscriminate fishing. Animals such as hammerhead sharks, giant rays and dolphins are all endangered in West African waters alone[6], and turtles, dolphins and whales are caught in nets intended for tuna in the Coral Triangle.

The global trend towards overfishing is made worse when you account for illegal fishing practices. In fact, some of the worst impacts on the ocean are caused by illegal, unregulated and unreported fishing, which is estimated to garner up to $36.4 billion each year.[7]

While super trawlers have been temporarily banned in Australia due to their catastrophic impact on marine life, they roam the oceans of the world largely unhindered. For many, their practices demonstrate no responsibility or respect for fish levels or the collateral loss of marine life. If this approach to fishing were left unchecked, we would see depleted fish stocks all around the world.

The global organisation MSC (Marine Stewardship Council) works to manage fisheries to encourage healthy fish stocks and avoid overfishing. I've been fortunate to witness the honourable work of the MSC, as I have worked with them for the last six years, and know firsthand the vital role they play in managing fisheries to encourage healthy fish stocks and avoid overfishing. Sadly, not all fisheries around the world subscribe to their policing – it's not mandatory – but those fisheries that do have an ethical, environmental and ecological commitment to fishing sustainably get benefits from the MSC. To be accredited by the MSC, the fisheries must follow guidelines and endure constant monitoring to ensure that the fish species are remaining resilient. The health of global fish stocks is constantly managed and reviewed to ensure threatened species are returned to safe levels.

Farmed fish have received mixed press in Australia. As in farming on land, the health of the marine life is highest when the living, feeding and breeding conditions most resemble that in nature. Detractors cite overcrowding of the fish pens and poor living conditions due to pollution from fish waste and uneaten food as the main problems associated with fish farming. But some in the industry address these problems by placing pens in deep water, giving their fish plenty of room to move by stocking fish at a low density and installing video technology that monitors any feed pellets that make it to the bottom of the pen, which then communicates to the automatic feeders to release fewer food pellets to ensure less wastage and avoid a build-up on the ocean floor. Fish farmers who are environmentally responsible will move the pens on and leave a site fallow to allow the seabed to regenerate.

I've spent time on the pens out in deep water in southern Tasmania and seen the conditions the fish live in. The particular salmon pens I've visited are huge, with the fish occupying only 1 per cent of the total space. The pens are located in open water, exposed to current, swell and the passing of nutrients. The salmon swim in shoal formation as they would in nature.

Another common claim in the farmed fish debate is that fish are fed colouring to ensure their flesh is the same as it would be in the wild. Again, whether a farmer does this or not comes down to their methods and ethos. I personally have spent time with farmers who categorically don't do this, but instead design their fish-feed to mimic what the fish would eat in the wild. Mimicking nature is the art of sustainable farming. So for me it's not an argument about wild or farmed, it's a discussion about the ethics of the farmer and which food system to support – intensive or regenerative. One supports the ecosystem and animal welfare, the other doesn't.

In many ways, sustainable fish farming employs similar principles as sustainable land farming: broadly, both methods work with nature, not against it. There are, however, a wider range of variables in fish farming, and it becomes our responsibility to do our homework and work out who are the best seafood producers in their categories – who ticks the boxes for animal welfare and environmental responsibility.

We have to be our own food detectives and support the right food system; it's not just a matter of farmed versus wild. Wild fish has MSC as a recognisable gold standard, and farmed fish has its equivalent: the Aquaculture Stewardship Council (ASC). This makes life a little easier when shopping for seafood, allowing one to be secure in the knowledge that purchasing ASC or MSC seafood will be supporting sustainable systems.

Look out for the ASC and MSC labels when shopping for seafood or ask your local fishmonger. In the supermarket, you'll see a blue tick if it's MSC accredited and a green tick if it's recognised by the ASC as responsibly farmed.

OTHER ETHICAL MEATS

The UK market can lean on alternative sources to meet the increased demand for protein. Throughout the UK there is an abundance of wild game, including venison, rabbit and pigeon. Without management, numbers of these species would spiral, negatively impacting on woodlands, crops and other wildlife. Culls are essential, which is why wild game is a truly sustainable meat source. Game is also delicious and has many nutritional benefits. You can ask your local butcher or check online for meats you can't find in the supermarket.

Venison

Deer numbers in the UK have never been higher. The six free-roaming British species total well over 1 million animals. Protection measures, such as fencing, are one way to reduce deer damage to woodland and farmland, but they need culling to keep the population under control. Wild venison is thus highly sustainable. If you can't find wild venison, farmed venison is still free range and grass-fed. Gram for gram, venison contains less fat than a skinless chicken breast and it has the highest protein and the lowest cholesterol content of any major meat.[8]

Rabbit

Eating wild rabbit makes good sense: since they are part of the natural environment, they put no additional strain on the earth's resources. Their free-ranging lifestyle and wild diet make for healthy, flavoursome meat.

Pigeon

Wild wood pigeon has a rich gamey flavour. Wood pigeons are predominantly birds of the countryside and can be pests to farmers and gardeners – therefore pigeon is a very sustainable meat. They are shot all year round so it is available fresh throughout the year.

THE ETHICAL ARGUMENT

Having worked in the health space for fifteen years, I know all too well the differences of opinion that exist in relation to what constitutes a healthy diet. From carnivores to fruitarians, everyone has a position on what they will allow themselves to consume. Some even relinquish the desire to eat physical food and embrace a 'breatharian' existence. Certainly makes for inexpensive and fuss-free dinner parties!

Everyone on this planet is entitled to choose what they consume, and with a growing vegan trend it's apparent that more and more people are giving up meat. It makes me wonder what is driving this trend? Could it be the proliferation of anti-meat documentaries on Netflix? Films such as *Cowspiracy*, *Earthlings* and *Food, Inc.* undoubtedly make people question the decision to eat meat, shining an ugly light on intensive farming, where animals are uncomfortable, crammed in small spaces and fed unnatural foods.

As a meat-eater I'm pleased that documentaries of this nature are out there for the world to see, if for no other reason than that they put the Western industrialised food system under the microscope. We do have to be reminded, however, that these shocking documentaries are not indicative of all farming, but that they go behind the scenes of a particular strand of farming – one that doesn't have your health or the health of the animal and land in mind.

The abundance and availability of food, including meat, in the Western world contributes to unconscious eating, whereby the shopper, diner, chef or home cook spares little to no thought about where that meat has come from. How it got on your plate, or how it got to your supermarket aisles, are important questions to ask yourself. Farming employs thousands of people, occupies enormous stretches of land and is integral to our existence, but for most part it's all done out of sight . . . especially for those of us who live in cities. Considering it's largely out of sight, perhaps it's understandable that many make the assumption that all farming is conducted in the way shown in those shocking docos.

The lack of comparison and context can fail to give consumers a true understanding of the whole industry. This can polarise people's opinions, which makes it harder to rationalise or reason with them. The bottom line is: you can't deny that an animal has been killed in order to provide meat, and if that guides your decision not to eat meat, then great. For me it's about choosing producers who have treated the animal humanely, feeding them natural foods and allowing them to move about rather than stay in cramped pens. I've visited Farmer Mick's farm numerous times and have witnessed firsthand cattle grazing in the lush pastures, cooling themselves in the dams and roaming as a herd, and it's that type of farming and produce that I support as much as I can.

At the end of the day it comes down to personal beliefs and values – everyone is entitled to have their opinion. No-one has the authority or right to force their opinion on anyone else. But it is important that the decisions we make are considered, objective and informed.

BE THE CUSTODIAN OF YOUR OWN HEALTH

The safest and only way to know exactly what meat you're consuming is to buy it and cook it yourself. Eating out at a café or restaurant, it can be a little harder to distinguish the quality of the meat. Unless the café or restaurant is singing about their premium produce from every empty space on their menu, it's fair to assume that they support non-regenerative farming practices – because, let's face it, hormone-free, organic and grass-fed produce is currently more expensive. Cost is a huge consideration when curating your supply chain and businesses will always try to minimise costs to maximise profit.

Take a look at your local food court and guess how many shops are selling organic and grass-fed meat versus buying produce from intensive farming in a bid to keep costs low. Hell, the cost of a McDonald's Big Mac in the UK is around £3.40 – which wouldn't buy you many organic nectarines, let alone much grass-fed ground beef! The current food system is skewed to favour empty calories – McDonald's is a cheaper option than organic fresh broccoli or a grass-fed steak.

To ensure you're the custodian of your health, it's necessary to buy, prep and cook *most* things you consume at home with your own hands. After all, our health is determined by what we do most of the time. I'm not naive enough to suggest that from now on, everything you eat must be made by you at home with real, organic food, but if most (70 per cent, 80 per cent . . . 90 per cent) is, then you're setting yourself up for optimum health!

Here's a breakdown of some key foods that I enjoy and that support a sustainable diet:

Grass-fed beef	MSC sardines	Olive oil	Organic berries (frozen or fresh)
Organic pork	MSC tuna	Organic and ethically sourced coconut oil	Local honey
Organic lamb	MSC anchovies	Homemade nut milks	Local or home-grown fruit
Organic chicken	MSC swordfish	Organic coconut milk/cream	Local or home-grown veggies
Organic eggs	ASC salmon	Organic ghee	Local or home-grown herbs and spices

It's worth noting that everyone's starting point will be different too. If you're just at the beginning of your health journey, home-made food might make up 20 per cent of your daily calorie intake, or maybe you're already an ace at this who spends most of their time in the kitchen fermenting foods into their labelled jars, simmering broths and brewing kombucha. It doesn't matter where you are, it matters that you're taking steps in the right direction.

Key Takeaways

1. Start to peel back the layers of food production and investigate the origin of your food. Supporting sustainable and ethical food systems is better for the planet, our health and animal welfare.

2. When choosing fish, it should not be just a decision between farmed versus wild; there are more questions to ask – both have good and bad ambassadors.

3. We are lucky to have plenty of both native and introduced species to choose from, including venison which is highly sustainable. Through investigating food sovereignty, we can all make informed decisions about which food system to support.

Chapter three

Is veganism the answer?

A great deal of science has emerged over the past 100 years regarding what constitutes the best nutrition for human health. Some research has been tinged with indirect or direct bias, with industries popularising their foods – or, conversely, rubbishing their competitors' foods – in a bid to win the market share. Only 70 years ago, cigarette brands such as Chesterfield and Camel were using doctors, nurses and dentists to endorse their products, with claims that their cigarettes lowered anxiety and stress, and even that they were beneficial in treating asthma, foul breath and head colds. Thankfully, in the case of cigarettes, the truth revealed itself, and tobacco companies now have to meet stringent laws about displaying health warnings. I feel a similar fate awaits the sugar industry and the fast-food industry . . . but don't let me digress!

The fact is, it can be a minefield to find unbiased information on nutrition. A global fear of saturated fats as the cause of high cholesterol and obesity began in the 1950s, and the sugar industry has sponsored studies over the following seven decades to keep the finger firmly pointed at fat, keeping the focus off themselves. It has become a game of chess between powerful players in the industry.

The EAT-*Lancet* Commission, a group of 37 leading scientists from across the world, released a report in January 2019 arguing that we need to make drastic changes to our current food systems. In fact, they say we need what they call a 'Great Food Transformation'. In their report, they identify food production as the single largest cause of global environmental change, responsible for around a third of greenhouse gas emissions, and a whopping 70 per cent of fresh water use. They also note that the clearing of land for crops and pastures is the greatest threat to species at risk of extinction.

When you begin to unpack the EAT-*Lancet* study and its recommendations, though, there are a number of things that don't stand up. Most significantly, the study relies on epidemiological research which can be unreliable, instead of clinical trials, when recommending the comparative benefit of a vegan/vegetarian diet to promote good health and fight disease. Zoë Harcombe, PhD in public health nutrition, identified some of the key problems with the EAT-*Lancet* diet: it was deficient in many essential nutrients: it met only 67 per cent of our potassium needs, 88 per cent of iron, 22 per cent of sodium and only 5 per cent of our vitamin D requirements.[1] Furthermore, there is a comment in the report that says animal items can be replaced with plant options – in which case it would be lacking in B_{12}.

The protein recommendations of the EAT-*Lancet* study also seem to fall short. The paper suggests that 0.8 grams of protein per kilogram of body weight is adequate, but it is widely accepted that a broad range of the population require additional protein for body function and maintenance: for instance, for athletes it is recommended that 1.8 grams per kilogram of bodyweight is needed, for most women about 1.6 grams per kilogram and for the elderly about 1.5 grams per kilogram.

While EAT-*Lancet* recognises that animal foods contain the nutrients needed for growth and health, it instead proposes a diet based on plant protein sources, such as beans and nuts. As the nutrients in plants are less bio-available (less easily absorbed by the human body), you would need to eat a significant volume, which obviously means greater overall calories, and would still result in a diet deficient in B_{12}, which can only be found in animal foods.

The study also suggests that a third of daily calories come from carbohydrates in the form of corn, wheat and rice, and 14 per cent from unsaturated oils (such as soybean, sunflower or peanut oil). These products and all their derivatives are highly processed and are, to my mind, suboptimal for human health. Despite the EAT-*Lancet* study's leaning towards a more vegan diet, the recommendation for vegetable intake was poor – only 3 per cent of calories were advised to come from vegetables.

The proposed diet does not provide adequate nutrition for 'growing children, adolescent girls, pregnant women, ageing adults, the malnourished, and the impoverished', and even those not within these special categories 'will need to take supplements to meet their basic [nutritional] requirements', says Georgia Ede, MD.[2] So, not the perfect global diet after all?

Chris Kresser, best-selling author of *The Paleo Cure*, also notes that when you work out the ratios, the diet ends up being low in protein and moderate in fat and carbohydrates. (He comments that there aren't many natural foods with that profile: breastmilk and acorns are two that he mentions – not foods most of us consume regularly!)

[T]hat macronutrient mix of low protein and then higher fat and carbohydrate is a recipe for highly palatable

and rewarding food. So if you look at the foods that are on this list that fit that profile, there are things like chocolate milk, potato chips, French toast, waffles, ice cream, pancakes.[3]

It is worth noting that the EAT Foundation, who worked with *The Lancet* to generate this recommended diet, also launched the Food Reform for Sustainability and Health, which is a partnership of multinational corporations, including Unilever (who sell vegetable oils and meat alternatives), Kellog's (who sell cereals) and PepsiCo (who sell sugar-laden drinks) – certainly a few of these companies might benefit from people eating their vegan/vegetarian packaged products.

VEGAN IN SHINING ARMOUR

Saving the planet and being vegan are thought to be synonymous, much like alfalfa and sprouts. I've already challenged the notion that becoming meat-free is best for our health and the planet, but there has been a significant expansion in the vegan movement – a recent survey found that 3.5 million people in Britain had chosen a vegan lifestyle in order to reduce animal cruelty and reduce their carbon footprint[4] – so we need to seriously examine veganism as an option . . . and consider a modified version of veganism.

There's no question that we in the industrialised world consume too much animal protein. Generally speaking, we could all do with reducing the amount of meat in our diet and replacing that protein with leafy greens and the like. Consuming too much meat from inferior animals (industrialised) and/or highly processed meat products is not optimal. Although I personally eat meat, I prize the veggies on my plate. Protein, to my mind, should be the condiment, and when you make veggies the hero you're truly giving your body the right inputs.

It's not surprising that people across the globe are ditching meat in a bid to reduce animal cruelty, but does going vegan absolve us of that guilt? Professor Mike Archer from the School of Biological, Earth and Environmental Sciences at the University of New South Wales describes how the agricultural process of clearing land to produce wheat, rice and other staples causes the death of thousands of native plants and animals per hectare. This monoculture farming practice brought to the land by European farmers has resulted in the loss of more than half of Australia's unique native vegetation – all for the production of food. And most of the arable land in Australia is already being used, so if Australians want a greater amount of plant foods to satisfy increasing vegan/vegetarian diets, it will mean that even more fertilisers and pesticides will be used, and even more land will be cleared. But the damage goes beyond just the land itself.

To produce protein from grazing beef, cattle are killed. One death delivers (on average, across Australia's grazing lands) a carcass of about 288 kgs. This is approximately 68 per cent boneless meat which, at 23 per cent protein, equals 45 kilograms of protein per animal killed. This means 2.2 animals killed for each 100 kilograms of useable animal protein produced.

Producing protein from wheat means ploughing pasture land and planting it with seed. Anyone who has sat on a ploughing tractor knows the predatory birds that follow you all day are not there because they have nothing better to do. Ploughing and harvesting kill small mammals, snakes, lizards and other animals in vast numbers.[5]

The death to sentient animals doesn't stop there though, the greatest loss of life is attributed to mice. Not only are millions of mice poisoned each year to keep them out of grain storage facilities, but grain production in Australia encounters a mice plague roughly every four years, with 500–1000 mice appearing per hectare. Farmers lay poison, which wipes out 80 per cent of these mice.

Professor Mike Archer does the maths. With beef, it was 2.2 animals for each 100 kilograms of protein, but for mice, he states that at least '100 mice are killed per hectare per year . . . to grow grain. Average yields are about 1.4 tonnes wheat/hectare; 13 per cent of the wheat is useable protein. Therefore, at least 55 sentient animals die to produce 100kg of useable plant protein.' That is 25 times more than for beef.

It is arguable, then, that red meat is a more humane and environmentally responsible dietary option, and this extends to other animal industries such as lamb and pork. When you consider the actual death toll of sentient beings, it does somewhat throw an ethical spanner in the works.

EIGHT TIPS FOR PROPER NUTRITION

It's an incredibly complex discussion, but ultimately any individual's desire to eschew meat needs to be respected. If you make the decision to be vegan, then it's wise to be diligent about ensuring your body is receiving all the right inputs. The following tips should help new vegans to navigate their way to good nutrition:

1. Avoid industrialised oils

Certainly limit, or avoid altogether, oils that are high in omega-6, as a diet with too much omega-6 has been linked with inflammation. These oils include sunflower, canola, safflower, soybean, vegetable and corn oil. These oils are also prone to becoming rancid. Instead, embrace a mix of avocado, walnut, olive, macadamia and coconut oils, as well as high-oleic sunflower oil.

2. Avoid 'white veganism'

Avoid a diet of white pasta, rice, white bread and highly processed foods. A diet rich in grains can lead to increased inflammation and disrupt the lining of your gut. Certain foods, such as grains, can cause irritation to the gut lining due to their natural pesticides (enzyme inhibitors), proteins or compounds, which make them problematic to digest. This in turn causes that low-level inflammation – hard to detect, but a potential setback for our health.

You should not underestimate the power of gluten as an inflammatory agent. About 1–2 per cent of the population have coeliac disease, and a further 30 per cent are non-coeliac gluten-sensitive folks, but the rest of us might not exhibit any intestinal disturbances when exposed to gluten. This doesn't mean, however, that we can indulge in gluten-laden carbs, as it can also have devastating consequences for the brain. We now understand the profound relationship between disruption to blood sugar and neurological conditions such as Alzheimer's disease and dementia. Having a diet high in carbohydrates and gluten can increase inflammation and the risk of neurological conditions.

A diet high in carbohydrates, and thus with elevated blood glucose, also promotes a process called glycation. This is characterised by an increase in blood glucose and a binding to proteins, resulting in two negative outcomes: the increased production of free radicals, which are potentially harmful to our cells; and the glycated proteins (those bound to sugar) dramatically increase the process of inflammation.

Furthermore, the antibodies that attack gluten also attack other proteins in the body, namely enzymes – which have similar characteristics to the gluten protein. These enzymes are called transglutaminase 2, 3 and 6.

Transglutaminase 2 is typically found in the gut, which is the reason people suffer from gut issues because of gluten – simply because the antibodies are attacking the gut tissues and breaking it down.

Transglutaminase 3 is typically found in the skin. So, when the antibodies attack these enzymes, people present with skin conditions such as eczema.

Transglutaminase 6 is typically found in the brain. When the antibodies attack these enzymes, then the integrity of the brain is diminished.

White foods are low in nutrient density. That's not to say you can't ever eat them; just minimise the amount and crowd them out with colourful, fibre-rich and nutrient-rich foods. Explore a variety of veggies and cooking techniques to ensure a broad range of nutrients is ingested.

3. Eat sprouted grains

If breads are your thing then being selective about what form they take can help. Breads made with sprouted grains are high in fibre and provide a broader range of nutrients, such as folate and vitamins C and E, than what you would find in processed white bread. Sprouting grains also have less phytic acid, which allows a higher iron absorption.

4. Eat real food

This applies to vegans, carnivores and everyone in between. Filling your pantry, fridge and ultimately your plate with fake foods – that is, highly processed and refined foods – is not sustainable for health . . . it's that cut and dried. Substitute those foods as best you can with real, unprocessed food.

5. Consider eggs

Eggs might be on the no-go list for many vegans, but pastured eggs can deliver a significant hit of nutrients and certainly are a natural superfood worth considering. It goes without saying that an egg is an animal product, but no animal has suffered. I'm not referring to caged or barn-raised chickens, but rather truly free-range, biodynamic or organic chooks. If you can't find any reliable egg producers, then there's always the option of keeping your own backyard chickens.

6. Consider oysters

Oysters are perhaps also a contentious food source in the vegan community, for obvious reasons, but oysters could potentially be on a vegan's menu simply because they lack a central nervous system. Therefore, if your decision to not eat animals is hinged on their felt pain, then this bivalve critter could be an exception. Oysters are rich in vitamin B_{12} and zinc, which are two nutrients lacking in an exclusively plant-based diet.

7. Consider insects

Vegan or carnivore, I'm sure we have all swatted a fly, and I'll bet my month's wages that we've all squashed a mozzie . . . so, perhaps insects are worth vegan consideration. A recent trip to Cambodia meant the obligatory sampling of various insects, some easily identifiable, others less so. Over the years I've tried many 'unusual' critters, but what is unusual to me is pretty standard to someone else – I've tried crickets, beetles, ants and locusts. In Australia or the UK (where I grew up), insects simply don't feature on the mainstream culinary landscape. But they are a sustainable food source, and are eaten the world over, providing much-valued protein. This is such an exciting option that I'm going to give it more attention in just a moment.

8. Take supplements

Three supplements you might need are vitamin B_{12}, algal oil and protein powder. Vitamin B_{12} is crucial for the healthy growth and cognitive development of children and ongoing wellbeing of adults. Algal oil is a vegan version of omega-3 fish oil – which smells better and is more environmentally friendly than fish oil production – that is important for brain development. When it comes to protein powder, hemp rules the roost, containing all nine essential amino acids, with brown rice and pea coming in a close tied-second. Traditional powders are made from whey, an animal product, but many options these days are gluten and whey free, and high in fibre and antioxidants.

Don't tie yourself up in knots. While it's admirable to have a firm philosophy on nutrition, there may be times when it's necessary to deviate from this in order to ensure your body is getting all its necessary inputs. Having a little flexibility in your diet will create a nutritional cushion to fall back on. Being vegan 85 per cent of the time but permitting yourself the occasional hit of ethically sourced protein can help to alleviate the risk of any nutrient deficiencies. Try not to pigeonhole yourself to the extent that your health suffers.

Michelle Yandle on veganism

I was so happy to interview Canadian-born Michelle Yandle, a prominent nutrition coach who now lives in New Zealand. Michelle spent much of her early childhood and adolescence as an obese girl. By the time she was fourteen she had been on countless diets, with little to no sustained reduction in weight. She regularly experienced low energy and apathy. Michelle was also an animal lover. In time she became an activist, campaigning against animals in circuses and eventually supporting and working within the RSPCA. It wasn't long before Michelle decided to give up meat.

That was when the change happened. She went from being overweight to lean, and her energy returned. Naturally she began cooking more at home, as her usual culinary haunts (KFC, McDonald's, etc.) were a no-go zone. Michelle became a proponent of the anti–animal cruelty movement, increasing her activism and stepping into veganism. For the next 27 years Michelle avoided meat as she periodically swung between vegetarianism and veganism. The rules and restrictions were clear-cut, as she adopted a zero tolerance for animal produce when following her vegan diet.

However, there came a point when her health declined. She recalls having very little energy and sleeping way too much for someone who was supposedly eating the right way. A blood test revealed low levels of vitamin B_{12}, zinc and iron. She began reintroducing eggs and cheese, but there was little improvement. Realising the minerals she was deficient in were animal-based raised some huge ethical questions, but she reintroduced animal products into her diet and regained her health.

Michelle's ancestry is indigenous Canadian, so she spent time considering what would have been on her ancestors' food landscape and how to bring that framework into her world. For Michelle it was about *quality* protein over quantity. She became invested in sourcing only ethically raised animals and created benchmarks that her meat had to reach in order for her to make a purchase.

Michelle says that for her it's not veganism versus meat but more about sustainable food sources and how to best support them.

MORE ABOUT INSECTS

A quick Google search for 'edible insect products' throws up a mixed bag of goodies. On the one hand you have ant candy and insect marshmallows and on the other roasted meal worms and loose-leaf tea with ants. These may be niche market products, but insects have the potential to occupy a significant portion of the protein market. A factor is the confronting nature of eating a bug or insect with its legs and wings impeding a smooth descent down the throat – but hey, deep-fry anything in spice, salt and coconut oil, and it'll taste bloody yum.

As our global population increases (exponentially over the next 50 years: by 2050, the UN estimates the world population will reach 9.8 billion), the conventional animal sources of proteins – chicken, cow, pig, sheep and fish – could be supported by insect production, particularly in the Western world. Sadly, most of us have an aversion to eating insects, but when looked at objectively it is no more peculiar than eating a lobster or prawn – both highly prized in the Western diet. Many nations of the world eat insects and regard them as a staple, and even a delicacy. Some Indigenous Australians forage for witchetty grubs. The larvae are sought after for their high protein content and are said to taste a little like almonds – but I haven't tried one, yet.

But if eating insects is out of the question, well I have news for you. There is a good chance that you are already consuming small amounts of insect or other animal matter in your food. The US Food and Drug Administration (FDA) have outlined the levels of 'natural or unavoidable defects in foods that present no health hazards for humans' and found that, for example, allspice powder averages one or more rodent hairs per 10 grams of powder and wheat will average 9 milligrams of rodent excrement per kilogram.[6] Even our beloved peanut butter may include one or more rodent hairs and 30 or more insect fragments per 100 grams. I strongly recommend visiting this online handbook to give you an idea of the tolerance for insects, mould, hair and excrement that can be in your foods – it's fascinating and a bit alarming, but it is the reality of the food we eat.

It seems inevitable, then, that the bugs and rodents that come in contact with our food may actually be in our food and knowing this makes the creepy crawly debate a little more complicated. For me, knowing that we are all likely consuming small amounts of insect matter (without any harmful effect) does not impact my food philosophy, as I personally choose to eat ethically sourced animal products, but it could be worth considering for those on a vegan diet. It could also open a door to accepting insects as part of the culinary landscape. Either way, I believe that insects will be an integral food source for the world's sustainable diet.

Studies have shown that many insects, like crickets, contain more protein pound for pound than beef. Crickets also contain a polysaccharide called chitin, which is a prebiotic and helps foster a healthy gut microbiome. I have included a few recipes later in this book using cricket powder – don't be afraid to try it out!

Edible insects are now being 'farmed' for mass consumption. From an ecological standpoint, farming insects is an alluring proposition, as the amount of land, water and feed required is negligible compared to cattle. Various insect rearing and processing enterprises are already emerging. Tiny Farms in California is leading the charge, offering Americans business opportunities to become insect farmers overnight. The start-up costs and associated risks are considerably lower for a prospective cricket farmer than, say, a cattle farmer.

To me, edible insects in the Western world are an opportunity to support the growing population in a sustainable and healthy way. However, simply adding insects to existing unhealthy products doesn't get the human race any closer to a health epidemic. I'm excited by the arrival of insects onto our food landscape and hopeful for the emerging industry. It's an opportunity to truly add value to food production and tick both the sustainability and health boxes, legitimately contributing to the ultimate sustainable diet.

THE PETRI DISH DEBATE

Such is the need for a revision of the current intensive farming systems that meat is now being made in a laboratory. While some chefs are disdainful of synthetic lab-made meat, we need to consider that it could be a legitimate contributor to the ultimate sustainable diet. The late Anthony Bourdain, celebrity chef, thought it a sad state of affairs when sustenance was put ahead of the magic of produce and the circle of life. He did also feel that we in the Western world waste a great deal of the animals we eat.

This is a sentiment I agree with and have raised many times throughout my books. For an animal to be raised, killed and butchered for human consumption requires a certain set of circumstances. These circumstances are a mix of physical, environmental and emotional, and to wholly respect the process the entire animal must be considered for consumption, not just the prime rib-eye fillet. It's vital that nothing goes to waste.

My last cookbook paid homage to this by including recipes for tongue, shoulder, liver, oxtail and cheeks. Many of us hold preconceived ideas on 'unusual' cuts of meat – for many people it has the 'ick' factor. The same attitude to insects is usually held about offal, but just as insects are eaten by millions of people around the world and are an integral part of their culinary landscape, so is offal. The less developed countries of the world would likely be horrified by our neglect for most parts of the animal. Their MO might not be health but rather survival, hunger and an aversion to waste, hence every part of the animal is utilised, including the feet, intestines, eyes and brains. Whether it's an eye or a beak, if it's cooked and treated the right way, it'll taste good. Anyway, back to petri dish meat . . .

So what is it exactly, and is it here to stay? Lab meat, aka clean meat, is produced by cultivating animal cells. No animals are raised or slaughtered in the process, yet for all intents and purposes it's 'real' meat. The technology is such that a sesame seed-sized biopsy (try saying that after a few wines!) taken from an animal supplies millions of cells. Place these inside a cultivator and the cells 'think' they are still inside the animal and grow normally into muscle. Advocates of synthesised meat claim that it's not just a substitute for meat, or even a meat alternative – it *is* meat!

The technology is not without its difficulties. One of the big challenges is to find the right liquid or medium in which to grow the meat cells. So far, this liquid has been foetal bovine serum, which is harvested from unborn calves. This, as you can appreciate, comes with a set of ethical questions and issues. But the bigger problem is that foetal bovine serum is not economical, due to the high cost of harvesting it. Research is now underway to find proteins in plants that can sustain cells to grow in exactly the same way as they would in foetal bovine serum. At the moment, they are running trials in oats, kidney beans, flax, pole beans, moringa and loquat plants.

Given that animal cells are grown in a cultivator and not within an animal raises an interesting issue – namely, the structure of the meat. Meat from an animal has a particular structure governed by limb length, placement within the body, attachment to tendons and muscles, and more, but these factors are absent with meat grown in a petri dish. Innovators might not yet be at the stage that they can replicate a sirloin steak or a T-bone, but advances are being made.

Lab-based meat is clearly a contentious product, but it's hard to challenge as a principle, considering it is born out of an imperative to feed a growing population without causing more animal deaths. Some corners of the food community are opposed to it, accusing it of not being natural – Bourdain even said it was the antithesis of everything he was promoting in the realm of cooking, foraging and hunting. For me it's an interesting innovation and a contribution to a sustainable food system . . . *if* done the right way. Looking at it objectively, lab meat isn't as 'natural' as grass-fed meat, using livestock which has lived a natural and healthy life, but as I've stated, *most* of the beef consumed in the world today sadly doesn't come from cattle happily grazing on lush pastures. So, is lab meat any less natural than intensively farmed animals, and could it offer a lifeline to those creatures born into intensive farming?

Interestingly, PETA (People for the Ethical Treatment of Animals) are supportive of lab meat. Their position is simply to eliminate animal suffering, and there's no doubt that lab meat does that, particularly when you consider some of the ways cattle are treated when raised for slaughter: their hooves may rarely touch grass, penned by steel fences and fed an unnatural diet to accelerate and maximise growth. The ethical hurdle is to find that plant-derived cultivating solution to replace the foetal bovine serum currently in use.

We are at the embryonic stage of lab meat production, with some large obstacles to overcome – for example, the current method is very costly with the first lab-meat burger reportedly costing $330,000 in 2015 (and I thought Sydney food prices were astronomical!) – but I've no doubt that our biochemists, food technicians and engineers will do it. The question is: can it be done in an ethical, healthy and sustainable way? Watch this space!

CAN PLANTS HEAR US?

Before I step off the veganism topic, I did want to throw one last thing into the mix. This whole chapter has been dedicated to unpacking what it is to be vegan and where the parameters start and end. Can a vegan include insects and bivalve organisms into their diet? Can they include lab meat? Does the whole vegan paradigm come crashing down once we take into consideration all the animals that are killed during the clearance and cultivation of intensively farmed crops? It's an incredibly layered discussion, and I'm just about to add another layer.

By definition 'sentient' is the capacity to feel, perceive or experience subjectively. I suggested that oysters could be on the culinary landscape for vegans because they lack a central nervous system and the ability to feel, perceive or experience subjectively. However, evidence has shown that *plants* may be sentient.

Studies are demonstrating that plants can make choices, show altruism and understand kinship, much like many animal species. Even as far back as Aristotle and Darwin, plants were acknowledged to have the ability to be aware of their surroundings and behave in response to stimuli and/or threats. Darwin, in his 1880 book *The Power of Movement in Plants*, proposes that a plant's roots act like a brain does in the animal kingdom.[7]

Professor Stefano Mancuso from the University of Florence discusses how plants move in accordance to their environment: they can flower, re-orientate themselves towards sunlight, and change their behaviour in order to sleep.[8] Professor Mancuso suggests that plants can detect and monitor up to fifteen physical and chemical parameters at any given time – now I feel lazy! Plants do this monitoring at the tips of their roots or the root apex. Here is where the plant communicates between cells – in other words, where there is an exchange of information happening. The root apex is only small, with a limited number of cells able to communicate, but the plant could have millions of roots and millions of apexes. So when you pull back from the single root, you can appreciate a complex network of communication designed to help the plant survive to its fullest potential.

Additionally, and fascinatingly, underneath a forest floor is an underground internet system – the mycelium. The mycelium is an infinite biological network of pathways that connect trees or plants and allows them to exchange information and share nutrients with each other, including carbon, nitrogen, phosphorus, water and hormones.

So, can we call plants sentient? Do their sentient properties create enough of a tipping point to prevent a vegan from eating plants?

The power of mushrooms to heal the land

Mushrooms are delicious cooked in thyme and butter, but they can also contribute to healing the Earth's wounds brought on by recent man-made actions. The intricate underground root system known as the mycelium not only helps fungi to communicate and share resources, but binds the earth and soil to combat erosion from poorly managed land. Mushroom and fungi occupy a staggering 25 per cent of the Earth's biomass. A quarter of *all* living organisms on Earth are mushroom or fungi, and this is due to the density of the mycelium.

But how else can mushrooms help the planet, you ask. Fungi help sequester carbon beneath the ground, taking carbon from the roots of aboveground plants and trapping it via the mycelium. Fungi produces a unique sticky protein called glomalin that also helps with the integrity and quality of the soil. The glomalin acts like a binding agent helping to prevent soil erosion and degradation. This alone is hugely beneficial for regeneration.

Mycelium can also break down the bonds in oil and diesel, absorbing it as food for growth. This has a multitude of benefits and applications, particularly in environments that have been damaged by spills or mismanagement. The mushrooms growing on the damaged land eventually spore and decay which attracts insects, and the insects then lay eggs. The larvae attract birds, bringing in seeds, and life returns to land which was desolate and toxic eight weeks previously.

Just as mycelium can be used to regenerate toxic land from petroleum spills or land mismanagement, it can also be used to intercept the toxic run-off, such as nitrogen and phosphorus fertilisers as well as pesticides, before these toxins enter water ways close to the property. Intercepting the contaminants with mycelium-packed porous bags is a Band-Aid solution to the problem, but a powerful one nonetheless.

Mushroom mycelium can also replace man-made products, such as Styrofoam, to lessen the effects of non-biodegradable landfill, and mushroom enzymes are also being employed in detergents – just another way that mushrooms have our backs, and Mother Nature's.

Key Takeaways

1. It's not as simple as a debate between vegan or meat diets – it's about supporting the most ethical, responsible and sustainable food systems.
2. There are deaths and harm to sentient beings no matter which food philosophy you uphold, so do your research.
3. Being open-minded to alternative food sources, such as insects, could lessen the demand on the intensive farming system.

Chapter four

Is keto sustainable for you and the planet?

Let me explain, for those of you who don't know, what the keto diet is. It is a low-carb, high-fat diet that results in ketosis. In short, ketosis is a metabolic state, wherein your body is predominantly using fat as its fuel source. By limiting total calories or carbohydrates, your body shifts from burning carbs to burning fat. Fat is metabolised in the liver and converted into ketones before being shunted out and made available to every cell in the body. Recording a ketone level of 0.5 mmol in your blood is considered being in ketosis. There are many health benefits of a ketogenic diet that I will discuss below.

A keto diet is not a rubber stamp for a sustainable diet – however, if you follow a keto diet that supports ethical, sustainable and responsible farming methods, it will be an excellent guide. As the keto diet is low in carbs (it's virtually impossible to eat pasta, rice or bread and be in ketosis) then there's less demand for those industrialised commodities such as wheat, barley and rye – therefore removing your support for those intensive food systems. When it comes to protein, it's up to you to support ethical farmers, and it's this that will determine whether your version of keto is sustainable or not.

I've been dabbling in keto for a number of years, and it's certainly a nutritional position that works well for me. Even when I'm not in nutritional ketosis I'm never too far from it (I'm only ever 100 grams or so of carbs outside of it). I've designed it this way because it suits my nutritional requirements, allows me to perform in the gym as I want to, and keeps me energised and healthy . . . plus I get to eat delicious fatty things. I'm able to swing in and out of ketosis very easily because the pendulum isn't swinging far at all. I have created a framework over the years, and the only tweak I make to my diet is the amount of carbs I have on any given day – and that's largely dependent on whether I've trained or not.

It works for me because I've taken the time to understand the *why* behind the principles and the mechanics of it, and I'm super-passionate about the *how* – the practical side, which of course includes cooking. In recent years I've written two books about the keto diet and its health benefits, along with 200 recipes – so I might be compromising sales when I say that there are certainly life-enhancing benefits from being in ketosis but what are we doing when we aren't in ketosis? If being healthy was easy, we'd all be enviable specimens; however, the myriad factors in our lives can pull us this way and that.

A term you're all familiar with I'm sure is the yo-yo effect. Quite often a well-intentioned plan goes out the window because the diet wasn't sustainable for that individual. With the emergence of the keto diet, I heard from and met countless individuals who jumped on the keto train, only to fall off days or weeks later. So spending two months in ketosis would be great, but what does your diet look like for the ten months of the year when we aren't knee deep in ketones? Our health is determined by what we do for all twelve months of the year, not the two months spent on a diet.

I believe the key is creating a 'diet' which is sustainable 365 days of the year and not one that the individual will give up on in a few weeks. It all feeds back into the master plan, which is the lifestyle you can adhere to consistently for the longest time. When I wrote the books in 2017, widespread uptake of the keto diet was yet to happen in Australia. I hadn't anticipated that so many people would be interested, let alone give it a red-hot go. Over the last two years I've seen and spoken to countless people who have transitioned from high carb to low carb and dabbled with ketosis. For most people it's a fleeting dance with nutritional ketosis – perhaps it's two weeks, four weeks or eight – but at some point, most folks sideline it. For them, being in ketosis is a one-off experiment, a type of 'detox'. So it's what happens after the two, four or eight weeks that will give our body the long-term feedback that determines health.

Let's assume someone dives headfirst into ketosis, does everything by the book and is recording in excess of 1.5 mmol every day for eight weeks – wonderful stuff. Once the eight weeks is up, does the pendulum swing all the way back to its original position – a position characterised by the consumption of refined and processed foods, high carbs and low fibre? If it does, the eight weeks spent in ketosis has been of little health value. Very often, however, people take on board some habits learnt from a high-fat, low-carb diet and are never too far away from ketosis.

HEALTH BENEFITS OF A KETO DIET

There are certainly a number of significant health benefits to be gained from a keto diet, such as:

- improved mood and cognitive function
- improved insulin sensitivity
- reduced inflammation
- neuron growth
- protected neuron health
- fat loss

Let's take a quick look at these benefits.

Improved mood and cognitive function

Being in ketosis will trigger a series of physiological responses, for example mitochondrial biogenesis – the growth of new mitochondria, the cells' power stations. It will also improve the function of existing mitochondria, ultimately culminating in optimised cell function and efficiency. Ketones have been shown to be the preferred fuel source for the brain and heart and have the ability to cross the blood-brain barrier (they're not hydrophobic), making them readily available to power your brain. Brain fog has been attributed to elevated levels of ammonia and lower levels of GABA (the 'chilled-out' neurotransmitter, which inhibits activity); ketones have been shown to increase GABA signalling and to help remove ammonia, helping to improve clarity.

Improved insulin sensitivity

Our ability to burn fat is largely controlled by our hormones. Elevated insulin impedes the burning of fat. When insulin levels are elevated, fat burning is dulled until such time that insulin returns to normal levels. Insulin resistance or insensitivity will result in chronically elevated insulin, making metabolising fat harder to achieve.

Reduced inflammation

Reducing or mitigating systemic inflammation is the core goal for myself and many of my clients. Assuming you've attained ketosis through 'clean' food then ketosis can inhibit inflammasomes, which are a part of the immune response which promotes inflammation. Lowering inflammation is the cornerstone to health.

Neuron growth

As I discuss in this book at length, it's not our inherited genes that determine our health but rather the expression of genes caused by lifestyle choices that accounts for 90 per cent of our health. We actually have the ability to grow new brain cells through a process called neurogenesis, which occurs when we produce BDNF (brain-derived neurotrophic factors), the fertiliser for the brain. There a few mechanisms that stimulate BDNF and being in ketosis is one of them.

Protected neuron health

Ketones elicit a protective response for the brain, which is highly significant in the fight against neurodegenerative diseases. As we age there tends to be a decline in the integrity of our brain cells. Studies have shown that ketones improve cognitive function for people with Alzheimer's, multiple sclerosis and Parkinson's. In fat, beta hydroxybutyrate (one of the three ketones we can manufacture) has been shown to reduce neuronal loss in animal models.

Fat loss

Increased fat loss is often the off-shoot of the pursuit of health. Being in ketosis will naturally increase satiety due to the foods you gravitate to, helping to normalise blood sugar and assist with cravings. To produce ketones, we need to 'liberate' body fat for metabolism (energy). It is this process, in combination with appetite suppression and lowered insulin that help to promote fat loss.

So it's clear to see that some life-enhancing properties are to be had when in ketosis. But there's also lots of health magic to be had even if ketosis isn't achieved. A diet that is low in carbohydrates but includes plenty of fresh produce has lots of value. It really comes down to the nutrient density of the foods you're consuming most of the time. The key to long-term health and longevity is to embrace a carb-appropriate diet (a term coined by Dr Cliff Harvey), which means you take sufficient carbs for your outputs and needs while simultaneously embracing a natural diet, free of refined and processed foods. In short, if ketosis is too hard to achieve and/or maintain, then having a little more carb flexibility might mean you can accommodate it in your daily life.

A point to consider is the quality of the food you're consuming on (or close to) a keto diet. The keto diet took the world by storm, but it wasn't long before the type of keto diet I prescribe got moulded, pushed, pressed and squeezed into a new version. Version 2.0 came with all the bells and whistles of an indulgent Western diet – it literally took all the unhealthy, fatty food from the Western diet and listed them as go-tos for keto. 'Dirty keto' was born. This approach ensures your macronutrients line up nicely, but pays little to no attention to your micronutrients. A quick internet search will reveal 'keto-friendly' meals full of processed cheese, whipped cream and ice-cream. Dirty keto is the intersection between the keto diet and the Western diet, marked by convenience foods and processed foods. Sure, it's possible to get into nutritional ketosis through v2.0, but you have to question the 'information' you're providing your body with: are the inputs the *right* inputs? Anecdotally I've heard of subscribers to this version of the keto diet scoffing KFC or McDonald's burgers (sans bun, of course).

To my mind, health should take into consideration the smallest moving parts of our bodies – cells. When you view personal health through cellular health – or specifically, mitochondrial health – you have to focus on the nutrient density of foods rather than just their calories. It's not that calories aren't important – they are, particularly if achieving a certain body composition is important to you – but it matters for your health where you're getting those calories from.

If I had a dollar for every time I'd heard 'food is energy', I'd be writing this from a comfy chesterfield rather than a wonky chair salvaged from a council clean-up. Yes, sure, food is energy – every food label comes with the number of kilojoules/calories indicating its energy value – but that's only half the picture. It's possible to maintain an 'ideal' body shape by keeping your eyes fixed on calories (energy), but at the same time be unhealthy.

Body shape is not a marker of health, and it's health I'm concerned with. Yes, you can have both . . . and that's ultimately what will happen if we supply our body with the right inputs. Health is a marker for health; we should look deeper than just body composition. There are subjective measures, including vitality, energy, mood, cognitive function, alertness, memory recall and focus, and objective measures, such as cholesterol (LDL/HDL ratio), red blood cell distribution, white blood cell count and iron levels. These measures are more reflective of your health than body composition.

I'm sure we all know people who have a body image we find desirable. I certainly do. For me, it's a strong athletic guy with muscular definition, vascularity and low body fat percentage. I personally know plenty of guys who fit the bill. Genetics plays a part, but I also know what they eat. The concept of food being anything more than energy is alien to them. For women, the aspirational body type is often a flat stomach, no cellulite, a thigh gap and thin arms. Again, this can be achieved via genetics and by monitoring energy intake versus output.

Body shape is *not* a marker for health, but being healthy will almost always result in a good body shape, so why not aim for the best of both worlds? You can have your cake – oops, I mean kale – and eat it too!

We are all geared differently and have different nutrient requirements, *but* no-one thrives on a poor diet. By refocusing the lens for health onto your cells and not your body shape, it's within us all to have health, longevity, vitality, energy, focus and alertness. In fact, I'd go as far to say it's our birthright. However, the Western diet and lifestyle have interfered with this relationship between food and health. We don't have to look too far back in our history to gain an understanding of how our diet and lifestyle has changed. We haven't always eaten highly processed foods, rich in carbohydrates, and nor have we led sedentary lifestyles. Our great-grandparents and all our ancestors before them would have been active and eaten only natural and organic foods.

Dirty keto is not sustainable for either personal or planetary health. However, eating keto, or close to it, in a manner that includes natural foods, organic where possible, with ethical meats, is sustainable for your health *and* the planet. As Michelle mentioned in her journey through veganism (see page 57), it really comes down to the *quality* of the food consumed.

Your body is robust enough to tolerate some indulgences from time to time, but if you give your cells good-quality inputs consistently, over a long period of time, you will thrive and be entitled to all the wonderful qualities associated with health.

Keto essentials

Some foods that are nutrient-rich and keto-friendly include:

Liver – Vitamins A, D, E, K, B_{12} and folic acid; copper and iron

Egg – Vitamin A, choline, folate, selenium, iodine, omega-3

Kale – Vitamins A, K and C

Bone marrow – Vitamin B_{12}, glycine, glucosamine

Garlic – Vitamins C and B_6, manganese

Ghee – Conjugated linoleic acid (CLA), vitamins A, E, D

Coconut oil – Monolaurin (antibacterial, antiviral and antifungal)

Turmeric – BDNF promoting

Sea salt – iodine, sodium, trace minerals

Seaweed – iodine, iron

Oysters – iron, magnesium, zinc

Berries – phytonutrients, polyphenols

Fermented foods – probiotics, vitamins A, B_1, B_2 and C

Cruciferous vegetables – fibre, vitamins A, C and K

The version of keto that I promote is most certainly sustainable for health, even if that means being on the fringe of keto and dipping in and out, or simply embracing a low-carb approach. Further, it can be sustainable for the planet if we choose foods that are responsibly farmed, fished and grown – in opposition to intensively farmed, fished and grown versions. It comes down to choices, and these are made every time you order food or shop in the supermarket.

As you edge towards the sustainable diet, some potent and powerful mechanisms are occurring. Every sip, slurp, nibble, crunch and bite is an opportunity to amplify your health. Let's explore how this is achieved.

EPIGENETICS

The conventional wisdom used to be that our genes determined our health and what diseases (if any) we might be susceptible to. This was called 'biological determinism'. In essence, the theory stated that the genes we inherited from our parents governed our resilience and longevity, thus setting our fate in stone . . . or in our genome.

The wisdom around genetics has evolved somewhat to accommodate the contribution of external factors on health. Currently it is accepted that external influences determine around 90 per cent of an individual's health. That's pretty significant, in anyone's books!

No longer should we accept the cards we've been dealt; we should be proactive in improving our health. The most effective and efficient driver for our own health is *us* . . . which harks back to my concept of becoming the custodian of our health . . . which is a fancy way of saying, take control!

External influences

Some top-line factors that will affect our health and wellbeing include:

- diet
- exercise
- sleep
- stress
- parental health at time of conception and delivery
- exposure to pollution
- whether you were breastfed
- alcohol consumption
- drug consumption

It's not that our environment and lifestyle (external factors) change our genes, but they affect the way there are expressed. Dr Christopher Wild proposed the concept of the 'exposome', the total sum of all the exposures that an individual has in a lifetime – from the first food they eat and the air they breathe as a child, to their lifestyle choices and social interactions – and how those exposures relate to health. Some exposures can leave a legacy, but it might not be felt for years or even decades.

I love Chris Kresser's explanation of epigenetics:

. . . a better analogy for genes might be a script for a theatre production or film. Our genes are like the script, and the exposome and epigenome are like the production and performance. The script of Romeo and Juliet *doesn't change from one production to the*

next, but how it is produced and performed can vary dramatically depending on the director, cast, crew, set design, costumes, and other factors. If a script is terrible, even a great performance can't save it. On the other hand, the best script in the world won't matter with a terrible production.[1]

Identical twins offer researchers the clearest insight into the role of epigenetics. Identical twins share the same gene sequence, so according to the old wisdom they should have identical health outcomes. However, this is rarely the case. Twins studied on epigenetic profiles reveal the extent to which lifestyle and age can impact upon gene expression, that is the process by which the genetic code of a gene instructs proteins to carry out their particular function. Manel Esteller of the Spanish National Cancer Research Center in Madrid found that 35 per cent of twin pairs had significant differences in DNA expression, finding that older pairs of twins were more epigenetically different than twin pairs of younger age. The analysis also found that twins who spent more time apart across their lives had greater epigenetic differences, suggesting that external factors (such as diet, exercise, smoking or drug use, exposure to pollution) can have a significant impact on how your genetics present.[2]

So variability in gene expression is clearly the result of environmental factors – exercise, diet, sleep, stress and so on. Knowing that external factors are the biggest driver of health and resilience to disease is comforting for most of us. But if you're reading this for the first time and feeling panicked because of exposure to pollutants, chemicals or just having not looked after yourself properly, try not to be alarmed (remember, we are robust organisms) but use this information to shape your lifestyle and environment. Change your habits and behaviour, and improve your existing environment as best you're able – perhaps by travelling a less polluted route, flipping your car air-circulatory system to 'closed' or working from home more often. Any positive change is an amplification of your health.

Stress

Stress is sadly part and parcel of the Western lifestyle; it's certainly present in my world. As I find new wisdom with age, I try to be less affected by stress . . . oh and my incredibly supportive wife is always there to peel me off the ceiling with her calm and bulletproof resolve. I often think she should write a book on managing stress, but that's a separate conversation.

Stress is one of the key external factors that can affect your health. Is there anything you can do to mitigate, reduce or minimise the amount of stress in your day? You could try using breathing techniques or not bringing work home with you, to create a clear demarcation between work life and home life. Again, stress is probably an inevitable part of life, but it's how we manage it that will govern its magnitude and the impact on our health.

Although it may take decades to make itself known, your health will be determined by what you do consistently over the greatest period of time. Understanding the risks and threats, as well as ways to improve health, can help to improve the long-term health of not just you and me but our community and the rest of the Western world. The power of a united force cannot be undervalued.

Junk food

It is possible to take control of your own health. Perhaps the biggest lever we have is nutrition. We eat several times a day, and every time we do, we send a specific code of information to our body. Unless we are working in an asbestos factory or smoking two packs of cigarettes a day, it's feasible to suggest that the food we eat has the biggest impact on our genes, health and longevity. This is great news. If epigenetics accounts for 90 per cent of our health-destiny, then nutrition surely accounts for at least half of that. Nutrients, minerals, trace elements and vitamins found in our food are the keys to good health.

Just as you want to make a good impression when you first take your new partner to dinner at your mum and dad's, you want to impress your body with food. To do that, you need to eat good-quality food. It can be a minefield when eating out or grabbing food on the go – your favourite café or restaurant will not (with a few exceptions) have your gene expression at the core of their decision-making. Most high-street cafés use cheap ingredients and cook them using fat, sugar and salt – the trifecta for taste, but not for positive gene expression. Monocropping, intensive farming and huge agri-business have facilitated the low cost of items such as sugar, wheat and corn. This in turn makes these items appealing to manufacturers, retailers, cafés and restaurants. Hence it is not surprising to see baked goods, confectionery, bread, pastries and lollies feature in the Western culinary landscape. In fact, so widespread are these items that they occupy 95 per cent of the shelf space in our supermarkets.

So if we can't rely on supermarkets, manufacturers, cafés and restaurants to take care of our health, who can we rely on? Ourselves! The only bulletproof method to impress your body is to prepare your own food each day and become the custodian of your own health.

Being young and active isn't an excuse to eat low-nutrient food. Junk food is giving your body information that leaves a mark and can manifest years later. Walking through the streets of my local beachside town I see a flurry of kids milling around after school. It saddens me to see Slurpees and packets of Oreos in their hands. The kids aren't to blame; the finger should be pointed at manufacturers, enticing kids and parents into thinking that the products they sell are healthy. We have a brand of breakfast cereal in Australia which has aligned itself with the national ironman competition. There's absolutely no doubting the physical prowess of an ironman/woman, but to have a breakfast cereal which is marketed as the breakfast for champions is misleading. It lulls kids and parents into a false sense of security. A bowl of Nutri-Grain, together with the suggested cup of skim milk, provides nearly 60 grams of carbohydrates, with little fibre to stall the glycaemic response. It is not the best start to the day for our wannabe ironmen/women.

LOOKING AHEAD FOR OUR KIDS

Little Timmy runs around all day at school and on the weekends. There is no obvious evidence that his diet is suboptimal. He is lean and energetic. He loves KFC and Ben and Jerry's ice-cream, but due to his activity levels displays no obvious evidence of his poor diet. As discussed earlier, body shape has very little bearing on health. Timmy's diet is not giving his body the right inputs, which may leave a lasting mark on his health. He is not necessarily destined for a short and diseased life; as he gets older he may become more conscious of his health. Timmy's long-term health and longevity will be determined by what he does over the longest period of time.

As a dad of two boys I'm well aware of the reward mechanism and how effective it can be to use positive reinforcement, but given the addictive nature of sugar, we have to ask the question: are we doing the right thing by our kids if we always reward them with sweet treats? That's not to say we can't use rewards, but we should be mindful of what the long-term effects may be. Every parent wants their son or daughter to be the happiest, shiniest, healthiest versions of themselves, so let's facilitate this for them while they are in our care. We should endeavour to set them up for health and longevity by imprinting as much positive coding as we can and start the epigenetic-ball rolling in the right direction.

Speaking to our kids when they are young about where food comes from is a really important piece to the puzzle. For them to understand food sovereignty and how food is grown or produced is the foundation to understanding the importance of supporting ethical food practices whenever possible when they are a little older. For there to be a strong swing back towards growing and producing food with compassion, it will require the next generation to be clued up. The last 100 years has seen a radical change in food systems through massive industrialisation and technology, and sadly this has squeezed out good animal husbandry and connection to the environment. It's up to us and our kids to push for more change.

Key Takeaways

1. Ninety per cent of our DNA expression, so ultimately our health and wellbeing, is determined by epigenetics – that is external factors, such as exposure to pollution, and our behaviours, such as exercise and drug use.

2. Out of all external factors, our diet has the biggest influence – so it is important to consistently make good food choices.

3. A keto or low-carb diet can be sustainable for human health and for environmental health, if you choose quality produce.

Chapter five

Daily rhythms

A growing body of research indicates that it matters a great deal *when* we eat, not just *what* we eat. It affects our biological clock, which determines when we wake up, when we go to sleep, and how our energy ebbs and flows in the time between. When we talk about sustainable diets, we're usually talking about growing and eating sustainably produced food, but there are other ways to look at it. For me, a sustainable diet is also one you can stick with and that will keep you feeling good over the long term – and that means a diet that works with your body's natural rhythms, not against them.

THE CIRCADIAN RHYTHM

There's a reason we feel energetic during the day, start to tire in the evening and sleep during the night. It's all down to the circadian rhythm – the natural, internal process that regulates the sleep–wake cycle and repeats roughly every 24 hours.

Many of our bodily functions peak at certain times of the day or night.

During the day:

- we experience high alertness, making us ready for the challenges of the day
- bowel movements occur
- cortisol rises, to prime our bodies for activity
- melatonin declines, to allow for wakefulness
- muscle tension increases
- we have better glucose regulation, to maintain energy metabolism throughout the day.

At night:

- repairs are made to the gut lining and skin
- growth hormones rise
- saliva production slows
- memories are consolidated
- melatonin rises.

A robust circadian rhythm is necessary for wellbeing, and when it's disrupted the effects can be significant. You may have experienced this if you've ever stayed up all night or travelled across time zones. It can disrupt your regular bodily functions, including digestion, sleep and defecation. It's well established that those who suffer chronic disruption to their circadian cycle, such as shift workers, are at higher risk of many serious health problems, including several types of cancer, cardiovascular disease and arthritis.[1]

Our diurnal nature was much more distinct in our ancestors. Pre-industrial humans had fewer disruptive factors to contend with. Their biological clocks were in tune with the 'nature clock'. Waking coincided with sunrise (there was no point waking before the sun came out), their muscle strength and mental alertness was at its best during the day (perfect for hunting and gathering), and as the sun went down their biological clocks pulled all the necessary levers to ensure they were prepared for sleep.

Sunlight (blue light) is picked up by a protein in our eyes called melanopsin. This inhibits the production of the sleep hormone melatonin. But as light diminishes, melatonin production begins to crank up, triggering a cascade of physiological responses that prepare the body for rest and rejuvenation. We have evolved to coordinate our bodies with the cycles of the day to optimise performance, alertness, survival and health.

Many modern technologies and behaviours interfere with our biological clock. This has an impact upon our health, both immediately and in the long term. Exposure to artificial lights, whether at work or at home in front of a computer or phone screen, is enough to disrupt our circadian rhythm. I know that whenever I've travelled to the outback for a few days I've found an overwhelming urge to sleep once darkness falls because there was almost no artificial light to trick my body into thinking it was daytime. The abundance of artificial light sources coupled with insufficient exposure to natural sunlight – a product of the Western lifestyle – is a recipe for ill-health. Too much indoor life can result in insomnia and not feeling refreshed in the morning. This can lead to migraines, irritation, depression and anxiety.

Your Daily Rhythm Checklist

There are strategies to help you tune your circadian rhythm, and some checks you could carry out:

- Are you having breakfast or drinking coffee at the same time every morning?
- Do you finish eating your evening meal two hours before sleep?
- Do you watch TV or look at a computer within two hours of going to sleep?
- Do you get sun exposure during the day?
- Do you feel rested in the morning?
- Do you sleep with the light on?
- Are you getting seven or more hours sleep a night?
- Are you anxious?
- Do you have reflux?
- Do you feel alert during the day?

If you feel like there's room to improve, then adjusting your habits and routines could help you achieve your health goals.

WHEN TO EAT

Knowing when to eat is a great asset on your way to taking control over your health. Although our circadian rhythm is influenced by the cyclic nature of day and night, we can influence our clock – positively or negatively – by our habits. For example, if your daily ritual is to eat breakfast at 8 a.m. right after waking up, then your body primes itself for this, first preparing for waking by raising body temperature and cortisol, then by secreting insulin and priming the digestive enzymes to ready your stomach for food. Your body becomes accustomed and schedules these processes to happen according to your routine.

When habits are broken then this sequence gets interrupted, like when travelling across time zones. An experiment by PhD student Jeff Plautz stumbled upon the understanding that the circadian rhythm of a fruit fly wasn't controlled by its brain but rather by each organ in its body.[2] This formed the basis of the work of Dr Satchin Panda, a professor at the Regulatory Biology Laboratory at the Salk Institute in California.

Dr Panda has recognised that each process of the body operates in a cyclic manner, and that each organ performs its roles at different times and tempos, and conducted experiments on mice by giving them food during the day when they would ordinarily be sleeping. Despite being nocturnal, within a short period of time the mice had reprogrammed themselves to wake just before food became available, before returning to sleep post-feed. What was most interesting in this experiment was that the liver function of the mice stepped up. Rather than being in the rest and restore phase of its cycle, liver function increased to process the food.

Fortunately, most of us are creatures of habit so we are rarely challenging our own clocks, but this next bit is really important, so pay close attention: our body needs the full range of a cycle to function optimally – it needs to be 'ON' and it needs to be 'OFF'. Your breakfast at 8 a.m. is not only a cue for your digestive system to turn on for the day but it's a cue to begin its cycle. Imagine that your digestive enzymes are shift workers that clock on at 8 a.m. and can work optimally for a further 8–10 hours, after which time they clock off – then you're in the 'OFF', or the rest and restore, phase.

Basically, your entire digestive system is doing shift work. Every time you eat, the process of digestion, absorption and metabolism takes a few hours to complete, even if it's just a snack or a nibble. After roughly ten hours of being 'ON', the gut and metabolic organs won't entirely shut up shop but their efficiency slows down, as they are not geared to run 24/7.[3]

TIME-RESTRICTED EATING

Eating within an 8–10-hour window corresponds with your own body clock to ensure the best health outcomes. Dr Panda warns that once we step outside this window for any length of time, our health is adversely affected. Snacking or eating meals outside of the optimal eight to ten hours promotes a fat storage mode. He explains that when you eat something, the pancreas releases insulin to help absorb sugar from the blood and tells your organs to convert that sugar into fat. This happens for two to three hours after each time you eat, so constant snacking is telling your body over and over to create and store fat.

> *Only after six to seven hours of not eating does our body begin to start burning some fat. This is the critically important aspect of time-restricted eating: to stop feeding the engine that is your body and let it run on the fuel it already has. This is the only way to prevent or reverse weight gain and, ultimately, obesity.*[4]

When the feeding window elongates and is more in the region of 14–15 hours, then it's more likely to promote insulin insensitivity, making the body work harder to regulate blood sugar levels, and be detrimental to muscle mass preservation. With the implications for insulin sensitivity, fat storage and muscle mass, you can quickly see how eating outside of the optimal 8–10 hours can be impeding your health goals.

It's certainly worth some consideration as I've had success with my clients simply by curtailing the feeding window. Ninety per cent of my clients come to me having tried various diets or health strategies but have plateaued and are looking for that missing piece to the puzzle. Restricted feeding is often the missing piece. Working with my clients I typically start with the quick and easy wins that we can implement straight away. Depending on a person's starting point, changing their feeding window can have profound results.

To help you prevent snacking when you first try to change your eating window, try a high-fat diet. Fats and proteins make you feel full and help to reduce cravings – both powerful tools when trying time-restricted feeding. Be aware that your digestive shift workers clock 'ON' when anything other than water is ingested . . . which includes coffee . . . even if it's black.

If you can manage to restrict your feeding window to eight or less hours of the day – when the fast hits sixteen-plus hours – then the magic really happens. Fasting triggers certain physical processes and improves mental clarity. For instance, fasting helps to promote the manufacturing of ketones. Being in ketosis not only provides your body with an alternative fuel source but inhibits inflammasones, helping to keep inflammation at bay, and promotes mitochondrial biogenesis and neural biogenesis, the growth of new neurons.

Essentially, fasting will promote a cellular process called 'autophagy'. Autophagy allows the cell to rid itself of any dead cell components, dead or dysfunctional mitochondria and toxins. Time-restricted feeding gives your body the time and space for autophagy during the 'OFF' time – or when the 'kitchen is closed'. Late-night food binges, or anything over your 8–10-hour feeding window, will compromise your cells' ability to detoxify. In addition to fasting in this way one or two times a week, I'd also recommend fasting for two to three days once every six months, once you have become accustomed to a low-carb diet approach and are metabolically flexible enough to burn fat efficiently.

Fasting can be done as often as it suits your lifestyle. Having an early dinner and skipping breakfast, then pushing through till lunch, is a really simple and effective way to notch up sixteen-plus hours of fasting. Having said that, fasting can be a challenge unless you're used to it. Start slowly and increase the length of your fasts as you become more comfortable. Practising a low-carb diet beforehand will help you through the process.

From a purist perspective, drinking anything other than water will break the fast, but coffee is a daily pleasure for many of us, and has been shown to be beneficial when fasting, to promote ketosis, fat burning and autophagy, so go ahead and enjoy a coffee or two – ideally a long black (my preference) or a coffee with an unsweetened nut milk will not be detrimental to your fast. Keep in mind that your digestive system will clock on as soon as you drink that first coffee, which will start your feeding window, and always monitor your caffeine dosage, as too much can have an impact on your sleep quality and level of anxiety.

SLEEP

In the interests of health and longevity, the importance of sleep cannot be overstated. It's often seen as a luxury, or simply something we do at the end of the day when we can't keep our eyes open any longer (watching the latest episode of a Netflix series . . .).

Many of us don't hold sleep in the high regard we should and the costs of sleep deprivation often go unnoticed, or are blamed on a bad diet or lack of exercise. Insufficient sleep has been linked to poor health outcomes, including obesity and diabetes, and is considered an important risk factor for these and other diseases. Although scientists have just begun to identify the connections between insufficient sleep and disease, most experts have concluded that getting enough high-quality sleep may be as important to health and wellbeing as nutrition and exercise.

Regularly sleeping fewer than eight hours a night increases the risk of developing a number of medical conditions. Results from several studies show that reducing sleep by just two or three hours per night can have dramatic health consequences, including weight gain, diabetes, cardiovascular disease and hypertension, impaired immune function and greater susceptibility to the common cold. Let's look at these in a little more detail.

Obesity

Several studies have linked insufficient sleep with weight gain. One study found that people who slept fewer than six hours per night on a regular basis were much more likely to have excess body weight, while people who slept an average of eight hours per night had the lowest relative body fat of the study group.[5] Another study found that babies who were 'short sleepers' were much more likely to develop obesity later in childhood than those who slept the recommended number of hours.[6]

Diabetes

Studies have shown that people who reported sleeping fewer than five hours per night had a greatly increased risk of having or developing type 2 diabetes.[7] Fortunately, studies have also found that improved sleep can positively influence blood sugar control and reduce the effects of type 2 diabetes.[8]

Cardiovascular disease and hypertension

A recent study found that even modestly reduced sleep (six to seven hours per night) was associated with a greatly increased risk of coronary artery calcification, a predictor of future myocardial infarction (heart attack) and death due to heart disease.[9] There is also growing evidence of a connection between sleep loss caused by obstructive sleep apnoea (when your breathing stops for up to a minute during sleep) and an increased risk of cardiovascular diseases, including hypertension, stroke, coronary heart disease and irregular heartbeat.[10]

Immune function

Interactions between sleep and the immune system have been well documented. Sleep deprivation increases the levels of many inflammatory mediators, released by your immune system in response to inflammation, and infections in turn disrupt homeostasis and affect the duration and quality of sleep.[11] While scientists are just beginning to understand these interactions, early work suggests that sleep deprivation may decrease the ability to resist infection.

The common cold

People who averaged less than seven hours of sleep a night were recently revealed to be about three times more likely to develop cold symptoms than study volunteers who got eight or more hours of sleep when exposed to the cold-causing rhinovirus. In addition, those individuals who got better-quality sleep were the least likely to come down with a cold.[12]

There is a strong argument to minimise or avoid disruptions to our internal body clock. Professor Eran Elinav and his team conducted experiments to identify the relationship between jet lag and health outcomes. The team collected bacterial samples from two people flying from the US to Israel, once before the flight, once a day after landing when jet lag was at its peak, and once two weeks later when the jet lag had worn off. The researchers then implanted these bacteria into mice. Mice receiving the jet-lagged humans' bacteria exhibited significant weight gain and high blood sugar levels, while mice getting bacteria from either before or after the jet lag had worn off did not. These results suggest that disruption of the biological clock can disrupt your gut bacteria and, in turn, increase the risk for such common conditions as obesity and imbalances in blood sugar levels. Mind-blowing![13]

It is true that a small percentage of the population can function on a few hours of sleep per night. A gene mutation called DEC2 allows those people who possess it to sleep fewer hours than us mere mortals. Instead of requiring eight hours for their body to rest and restore, DEC2 gene holders can do the same in four hours. Margaret Thatcher famously stated that she only needed four hours of sleep a night to function. Not that I'm likely to be asked at this point in my career, but I should flag that as prime minister I'd require eight hours of blissful sleep per night, thanks.

WORK ON YOUR SLEEP

I strongly advise you to exercise your sleep muscles and 'work' on sleep. There are number of strategies you can employ:

Sleep in a cool room (17–19°C). It's not always easy, but if you can manage it, keep the temperature down and you'll optimise your slumber.

Wear earplugs and/or an eye-mask. You can't always control the noise or lights coming from outside your bedroom but wearing earplugs or an eye-mask can certainly drown out some ambient noise and unwanted light. You could also try blackout curtains.

Avoid tech for the last two hours of your day. Try a blue light filter to prevent the blue light emitted by devices such as phones and laptops interfering with your circadian rhythm.

Have a hot and cold shower. Alternating between hot and cold water when you have a shower before bed will help to promote good-quality sleep. Shower at your usual temperature, then gradually add hot water to a point at which it is uncomfortable. Ensure your whole body experiences this temperature. Slowly turn down the hot water until there is only cold water running and expose your whole body to this. Raise the temperature again (if you can tolerate a higher temperature than before, do so). Then lower the temperature again and repeat six more times. Finish with cold water.

PAYING YOUR SLEEP DEBT

As evening approaches, our organs' internal clocks begin to synchronise to create the perfect conditions for sleep. Melatonin is secreted, heart rate slows and body temperature drops. In a perfect world, at this point we slip between the sheets and within 30 minutes we have drifted off, to enjoy uninterrupted sleep for eight hours (or ten for a child). That ideal scenario rarely occurs, however. When the actual sleep time doesn't match the required sleep time, a 'sleep debt' is incurred.

Again in a perfect world, our sleep should follow distinct cycles marked by quiet and active sleep, with one cycle including both phases. We typically experience three to five cycles per night, occurring every 90–120 minutes, although the initial cycles are relatively short and increase as the night wears on. Our quiet sleep is characterised by three stages: drowsiness, light sleep and deep sleep. During the first stage you begin to lose awareness of your surroundings. Your muscles relax and your eyes move from side to side. Light sleep, the next stage, is true sleep, as the body temperature drops and heart rate and breathing slow. This stage is characterised by spikes of brain activity, which researchers suggest is us consolidating memories. The third stage, deep sleep, is marked by low blood pressure and a cooling of the brain. It's during this sleep that the muscles which enable us to stand upright become paralysed, disabling us from acting out our dreams (which is lucky, because I have lots of flying dreams). All the stages are representative of 'quiet sleep', which will be followed by active sleep, or REM (rapid eye movement) sleep. During REM, some of our functions tick along at daytime speed, such as blood pressure and breathing.

If your partner doesn't snore or the kids don't wake you, you can rest and restore for eight hours each night. Even if nothing interrupts your sleep, the truth is that for many of us eight hours of sleep a night isn't going to happen – not while Netflix keep releasing enticing series after series, damn them!

Every time we fall short of the desired eight hours, we are put into a sleep debt. Sleep debt, as previously mentioned, is the difference between desired sleep and actual sleep. For us to perform and function optimally, we must repay the debt that we accrued the night before. This can be done by going to bed earlier the night following a poor sleep, or napping in the day (if you can). Weekends provide another opportunity to repay a sleep debt. I see this played out with my son, Tashi, who generally gets eight to ten hours of sleep on a school night but can easily get twelve-plus or more on a Saturday or Sunday.

But many of us fall short of the desired eight hours and rarely or never repay the debt. Think parents of a newborn baby, for one! The long and short of it is that sleep is essential to sustaining good health. If you are not getting consistent quality sleep, start to dissect the reasons behind that and develop a strategy for how to remedy it – or at least improve it. Sleep is a foundation to achieving health and longevity . . . and avoiding the grumps!

EXERCISE

It would be remiss of me to discuss a healthy lifestyle without talking about fitness and exercise. Training is in my DNA. For a long time it forged my identity; I was known as the 'fit guy' or 'the guy that runs a lot'. Those appellations made me feel good, but the reality was I was slowly ruining my body. I trained every day and trained hard, too. This set me up for injury – which eventually came in 2005 with a serious back injury. The bottom line was, the exercise I had been doing wasn't sustainable . . . which is ultimately what this book is about – finding the path to a sustainable diet and lifestyle.

Since I recovered from my back injury, my goal has simply been to be able to train whenever I want, which means staying injury-free. I still train a few times a week and train hard, but not to the point of compromising my goal or my health. To me, training is a mood enhancer more than anything. It allows me to feel positive, strong and agile. My typical week will include four or five gym sessions, a walk with my wife and one or two surfs. Before my injury,

I wouldn't want to leave the gym unless I was physically exhausted and drenched in sweat. Now I take my time and I've noticed the benefits of not flogging myself like I used to: I have more energy throughout the day, and my immunity is great.

For exercise to be sustainable and indelibly imprinted into your master plan, it has to be something you enjoy – simple as that. The gym isn't for everyone. Find a form of exercise you enjoy doing and can do regularly. That's not to say it has to be the same thing on each occasion, nor that it can't change over time, but it has to be pleasurable. I say this because fitness is not the sole path to health and longevity. Sure, it can contribute and add value, but nutrition and sleep are the biggest drivers. So let's assume your nutrition and sleep are on point. This allows you to relax a little with fitness and open the door to play and pleasurable pursuits. Exercise is simply the cherry on top, further optimising your health.

As I've mentioned previously, we can influence the genes that are expressed through epigenetics. Further to this, we can promote life-enhancing physiological processes as a direct result of nutrition and lifestyle choices. This is evident with exercise and its promotion of brain-derived neurotrophic factor (BDNF) – our own brain fertiliser. BDNF is stimulated when we exercise, encouraging the growth of new neurons, improving the function of existing neurons and the connection between neurons, as well as improving memory . . . strong enough reasons to exercise!

Exercise is also a fantastic mechanism for lifting one's mood, and if you're someone who likes to exercise in the morning (like me), it can really help set the tone for the day. Options for exercise can include 'blue' fitness – water activities like swimming or surfing – and 'green' fitness – land-based activities like bushwalking, cycling or playing football.

To me, surfing would be up there for mood elevating exercise – once you're out in the ocean, it's very hard to feel stressed about work or other issues. That's not to say your worries will disappear, but for the time you're paddling they fade into the background, and you are getting some daylight too, which we know will help your body regulate sleep. Surfing has also become a bonding activity for me and my son, Tashi, so I have a compelling reason to maintain my fitness.

The heightened mood from exercise will most likely have a positive impact on decisions made throughout the day – including nutritional choices around food. If you're feeling good about yourself as a direct result of exercise, you're much more likely to gravitate towards healthy foods.

A study published by the American College of Sports Medicine found that acute bouts of exercise were enough to increase mood in patients suffering from major depressive order[14] and exercise physiologist Simon Rosenbaum from The Black Dog Institute has been using exercise as therapy for his patients with depression and PTSD and has seen positive outcomes. A combination of 'blue' and 'green' fitness opportunities, plus strength training, has been seen to improve the mood and outlook of patients. It is less about the intensity of the exercise and more about actually being engaged and active. Even low-intensity exercises such as swimming and walking elicit positive outcomes.

As humans we are designed to move, and move often. Low-intensity activities such as walking form the foundation of our fitness and so we should engage in this activity several times a week. Much of this is taken care of with incidental fitness: shopping, gardening, etc. However, we are also designed to move our body in more explosive ways from time to time. These actions include pushing, pulling, squatting and climbing, so factoring in some of these each week is paramount to sustained fitness. Also include some heavy lifting (it's all relative – just do what is right for your body) and try sprinting once a week – it delivers a myriad of benefits.

70 %		20%	10%
Blue Fitness	Green Fitness	Lift heavy objects	Sprinting, high-intensity cardio
Swim	Garden		
Paddle board	Hike		
Surf	Walk		

The table above represents an approximate target of exercise intensities that you should aim for throughout the week.

MAKE IT WORK FOR YOU

Clearly there are a number of things to consider when optimising your health. It's important to have a nutritious diet, get enough sleep and exercise, and you should aim to feed within an 8–10-hour window.

When I'm working with clients, there's zero sense in making lifestyle recommendations without looking at their manner of living, day to day. What does their work week look like? What does their average weekend look like? Understanding these things gives me a framework from which to make suggestions for strategies to improve health, so step back and take a look at your habits and routines, and see where you could make adjustments.

As you make the changes towards reducing your feeding window, improving your nutrition and sleep, and increasing exercise, be sure your new routine fits into your lifestyle and meets your energy requirements throughout the day. Knowing the right information and hearing good strategies for change is important, but it won't amount to much if you don't employ patience, perseverance and planning. Taking small steps is the only way it'll work for you in the long-term and be truly sustainable!

Key Takeaways

1. Fasting for sixteen-plus hours is a great way to elicit some life enhancing properties. I recommend spending some time engaging in a low-carbohydrate diet before jumping in with both feet. Restricting your feeding window to 8–10 hours will sync with your digestive system's optimum efficiencies, which is beneficial to health.
2. Sleep is a foundation to achieving health and longevity, so work on strategies to optimise your sleep.
3. Fitness isn't the sole pathway to health, but it is the cherry on top. Invest in your nutrition and sleep, and then add some exercise which incorporates 'play' – only then will your health plan be sustainable.

Chapter six

Investing in your health

The fact that you're reading this book says a great deal. It means you're invested in your health, and probably in the health of your loved ones. Understanding the foundation of a diet is imperative to long-term success. Once you have established a framework, then you can customise your diet to suit you.

I've given many presentations on health and nutrition, and one of the most commonly asked questions is, what does my plate look like on a typical day? I always respond in fairly broad terms, because the food I eat reflects my budget, food availability, time management and preferences. For another individual to replicate what's on my plate wouldn't be true to him or her. It's through customising a diet to suit you and your lifestyle that you'll find the key to long-term adherence.

NUTRIENT-DENSE SHOPPING

Before you can cook you need to shop. Load your basket or trolley with fresh, unprocessed produce. Foods that were once alive – that is to say, meat, fruit, vegetables, and so on – should comprise the majority of your purchases. Live or real food is packed full of 'information' in the form of minerals, nutrients and vitamins, which your body needs in order to achieve optimal health. Giving your body the inputs it requires is fundamental to cellular health and longevity. Look for shellfish, fish, organic and grass-fed meat, cruciferous veggies, spices, poultry, eggs and even insects. Nutrient density will give you more nutritional bang for your buck and keep you satiated for longer. With the appropriate macronutrient split – optimum amounts of carbohydrate, protein and fats – it will serve to keep you feeling fuller longer.

There's a reason people experience the desire to eat again shortly after finishing a Big Mac. It isn't a case of gluttony; it's that the ingredients in the burger trigger a particular set of hormonal reactions that result in you being hungry sooner. So although a Big Mac is cheaper in the short term, the upshot is you'll be eating with greater frequency when compared to eating nutrient-dense foods. With the appropriate macro-split and nutrient density, you'll be eating less often – maybe two or three times a day – and snacking will go out the window. Grazing all day is a strange concept for humans and certainly wouldn't have been how our ancestors ate. We aren't ruminants (last time I checked), and eating throughout the day is not optimal for our digestive systems. Our digestive systems need the 'OFF' time to process food. If we give ourselves the right inputs, then health, optimal weight and longevity is in reach.

Investing in your health is worth it. But when your basket is brimming with fresh produce, organic eggs and grass-fed protein, you'll be hit harder in the hip pocket than if you bought processed foods. On occasions I've left a health-food store analysing the receipt, my eyes darting back and forth between it and my meagre box of goodies in the hope that the shop assistant got it wrong. 'Surely there's been a mistake!' I say to myself. If my bank balance had a few more zeros on it then I wouldn't blink an eye at the cost of organic fresh produce, but the reality is I have to budget. Now, I'm certainly no barefoot investor or financial wizard (my wife will testify to that), but my belief in the importance of nutrition justifies spending *some* of my hard-earned money on great-quality produce. When doing my grocery shopping, I run all my choices through a filter, which goes something like this:

1. Is it delicious?
2. Is it healthy for me?
3. Can I afford it?
4. Does it need to be organic?
5. Does it need to be grass-fed? (for proteins)
6. Does it need to ethically sourced?
7. Do I need to buy the best in the category?
8. Is it a brand I trust?
9. Can I shoplift it without getting caught?

The first eight questions are legitimate. Not all of the products I purchase are organic. I do have some non-negotiables around meat, fish, chicken and eggs – they have to be sustainably sourced and organic – but the rest is pretty much up for debate. Unless I'm at the farmers' markets or the organic health food store, most of the veggies, herbs, spices and other items I buy are from my local supermarket and are not organic. It's a trade-off, I guess. On the one hand my health is better, as I'm choosing fresh produce over processed and refined products, but on the other I'm unlikely to be supporting regenerative farmers by shopping at a big supermarket.

I can only hope that this book becomes a *New York Times* bestseller and I get to add organic veggies consistently to my shopping trolley! Until that time (and I've probably more chance of becoming prime minister), here are my recommendations for navigating shopping for health.

Buy cheap cuts

Western society prizes neat-looking prime cuts over others which are perceived as less desirable, so there's great value in shoulders, cheeks, shanks and bellies. I'd go so far as to say they are not only cheaper but pack more of a flavour punch. Another bonus is that the margin for error is reduced: it's harder to overcook a shoulder than it is to overcook an eye fillet. Growing up, I was served up an array of these cheaper cuts, as well as organ meats, and I loved them.

Purchasing cuts of meat which have the bone still in is another way to save your money. Speak to your butcher about cheaper cuts if you're unsure where to start.

Buy a Cow

Yes, you read that correctly. These are harder to shoplift, that's for sure, but it's more affordable to buy in bulk. Like any commercial exchange, it's more economical to purchase a complete item or product than it is to buy the individual components that comprise the whole.

There are initiatives that allow small groups of people to buy a whole cow. Ethical Farmers, a Sydney-based company, is driving community initiatives to help keep costs low. Their philosophy speaks my language: they offer lower-cost organic/ethically sourced produce, plus keep wastage to a minimum. The meat, fat and bone (an entire carcass) of a grass-fed cow is shared between eight participants, somewhere between 22–30 kilograms each. This might not be for everyone, but eating all parts of the cow, not just the prime cuts, provides greater nutrient density, and this community-style purchase is an ethical meat model. Participants can even visit the farm to see where their animal grew up.

Buy in bulk

As with the 'share a cow' scheme, buying in bulk either as an individual, as a pair or in a group can save dollars. There are plenty of bulk goods stores around Australia that offer a more affordable way to shop for oils, nuts, seeds and even household cleaning products. Many of the products sold are organic, or at least ethically sourced, but always read the label.

Avoid the middle aisles

As I've already said, stocking your pantry and fridge with nutrient-dense foods means fewer trips to the fridge and fewer trips to the supermarket . . . saving you money in the long run. Nutrient-dense foods may cost more upfront but they should improve satiety and reduce the frequency of eating. Purchasing cheap processed/refined foods from the middle aisles of your supermarket is tempting, but these items will more than likely spike your blood sugar (high GI foods), resulting in the need to eat more frequently. Processed foods are an amalgamation of cheap commodities (sugar, corn, wheat, stabilisers, etc.). They have little nutritional value and only drive metabolic syndrome by stressing your insulin sensitivity. Buying fresh over packaged is the sure-fire way to get nutrient density into your shopping trolley.

To take this concept a little further, you could look at a low-carb/
high-fat diet, which will increase satiety by normalising blood sugar,
increasing insulin sensitivity and normalising your hunger/satiety
hormones (look back to chapter four for more information about
the benefits of a keto diet).

Freeze

Frozen produce such as veggies and berries are cheaper than their
fresh counterparts and are nutritionally comparable. There seems
little evidence to suggest that there are advantages to buying fresh
peas (expensive) over frozen peas (cheaper). The same applies to
berries. If you see a price-reduced fresh-food item in your supermarket, such as a cut of meat or fish, you can always snap it up
and pop it in the freezer. It will save you money in the long run;
it's a no-brainer.

Make your own

Buying condiments and sauces off the shelf can be expensive, so
to save money you could attempt to make your own. This requires
time, admittedly, but it comes with a financial win and is much
more satisfying. Added to that, you can always improve on the
nutritional aspects of store-bought sauces. My wife and I recently
made our own hummus, which was super-affordable and didn't
include any of the cheap oils commonly found in dips. Keeping
chickens is another way to reduce spending; you are delivered fresh,
free-range eggs daily.

Growing your own herbs or veggies will help to keep costs
down. The scale of a grow-your-own operation is dependent on
the space you have, but even the most compact living arrangements
can produce a yield through ingenuity. If you're short on space in

your garden, you can add a window box of herbs or intersperse veg between your other plants and flowers. Growing 'up' by using climbing plants is another way to combat a lack of space – try cucumbers or climbing vines of tomatoes or squash.

Finally, companion planting is often touted for the benefit of cutting down on pest infestations, but it also serves to conserve space. Shade-tolerant plants benefit from being planted next to taller crops. For example, basil likes a respite from the hot sun and does well next to tomatoes.

Go to farmers' markets

To support a local market is to make a stand for sustainability. Farmers' markets are a hub for local producers and boutique businesses, and a magnet for the people who seek ethical produce. Yes, the foodstuffs can come with a high-ish price tag, but until the pendulum swings away from the intensive food system, that's how it's going to be. Economic principles dictate that if demand increases (and so long as it can be met), prices will fall.

WORK YOUR KITCHEN MUSCLE

Aim to cook most of the things you eat or drink yourself, that way you won't be at the mercy of a manufacturer or producer. Real food – broccoli, chicken, fish, spinach, kale, cabbage, eggs, etc. – doesn't come with a food label, it simply is what it is. However, refined and processed foods have been conjured up by manufacturers in order to lure you with flavour. More often than not this will involve jamming in weird and wonderful ingredients. Most manufacturers and restaurants operate in a commercial and competitive space, and so your health isn't a primary goal for them; they're more interested in maximising their bottom line and know how to do that by combining the winning ingredients (sugar, fat, salt) in the right ratios.

Becoming the next Jamie Oliver in the kitchen won't happen overnight but it can happen. Just as with any new skill that you're hoping to refine, it requires practice, practice, practice. There will be lots of trial and error – and a few disasters along the way – but we all learn from our mistakes. If this is the start of your health journey, don't try to run before you can walk; keeping your dishes simple and fuss-free will set you up for success in the beginning. I have included a number of quick and easy recipes for beginners in part two of this book (see Easy Moroccan Chicken on page 216, Sautéed Veggies on page 226, and Slow-cooked Lamb with Anchovies on page 187).

Craft a small collection of dishes and slowly refine them to your tastes and your kitchen. Follow a recipe, by all means. Over time you'll probably remember what ingredients are required for that dish and in what quantities. You'll most likely go 'off-piste' and modify the recipe slightly because you've learnt it's tastier with more/less fat, salt, spice, herbs or heat. Once you've replicated it enough times and refined it to your preferences, it's then yours to own. The repertoire of your dishes should include (but not be limited to) a couple of salads, some slow-cooked dishes and a curry or two.

Get excited about being in your kitchen. This might mean giving it a spring clean or investing in a new knife or chopping board. When I first met my wife, she was chopping with a knife that hadn't been sharpened for years (she was better off chopping with a wooden spoon, to be honest). Little things like a sharp knife can make a huge difference to enjoying a cooking experience.

In order to improve your health, you'll have to be creating yummy food – delicious enough to entice you back to the kitchen tomorrow, the next day and for the rest of your days. It might sound like an ominous task, but with some practice and perseverance, you'll be experimenting with new dishes in no time. Here are some really simple tricks, tips and hacks to lift your cooking and make you the envy of the neighbourhood.

1. HEAT

It might sound painfully obvious, but heat is really important to cooking. Selecting the correct heat and adjusting the temperature throughout the cooking process can bring out the best in ingredients.

Fire has been available to humans for hundreds of thousands of years, and the use of it sets us apart from other species. So integral is fire to us that in 2016 it was argued that our species is an 'obligate' fire user – that is to say, all civilisations depend on it in some form. Our relationship with fire is even written into our genes: researchers identified a genetic innovation, the 'AHR' gene, which seems to have made our cells 1000 times more resilient to the carcinogenic effects of wood smoke. Neanderthals did not possess this gene.[1]

No-one knows exactly when humans first learnt to make fire, but it was relatively recent – within the past 400,000 years.[2] Harvard biologist Richard Wrangham suggests that it was our ability to make fire and cook our food that allowed us to progress as a species. He explains that eating raw foods requires more time and effort and hinders cognitive development. Eating raw foods is not the most efficient method to extract calories and nutrients, as most of the raw food eaten goes undigested to the small intestine, where it feeds the trillions of bacteria – essentially, lost calories that could be used to fuel the brain. Cooked food, by contrast, is mostly digested by the time it enters the colon; for the same number of calories ingested, the body gets significantly more energy (30 per cent from cooked oats, wheat or potato starch, and as much as 78 per cent from the protein in an egg).

Cooking, which includes not only heating food but the mechanics of chopping, pulverising and grinding, performs some of the digestion process for us, therefore less energy is required of us to break down the food inside our bodies. During the heating process, animal and plant matter is broken down, including collagen and connective tissues as well as the cell walls of plants. Cooking frees up not only valuable energy but time too – consider the fact that the great apes spend four to seven hours a day just chewing their food, which has stifled their bandwidth for other things.[3]

Understanding how different foods react to heat is learnt through exposure, practice, and trial and error. It's important to treat foods in the correct way in order to enhance flavour.

How to cook meat

The temperature and cook time for meat will be determined by the cut of meat you're dealing with. Generally there are two types of meat: ones which respond well to intense heat for a short period of time, and ones which respond well to being cooked at a lower temperature over a longer time. When cooking a fillet steak, most chefs will suggest starting with a hot pan and cooking the steak for 3 minutes on either side, then allowing to rest for 3 minutes. Conversely, when cooking a beef cheek you'd cook for 3–4 hours on 140°C and allow to rest for 20 minutes. Beef cheeks contain more connective tissue – more gelatine and collagen, which requires a longer time to break down, whereas fillet steak is pure muscle fibre and requires a short cook time.

For cuts such as shanks, shoulder, brisket and ribs, you'll need to prevent the meat from drying out – an easy way to achieve this is to cook the meat entirely or partially submerged in liquid. Then create a closed environment, such as by using a crock pot or Dutch oven to prevent evaporation, or if you don't have either of those wrapping a couple of layers of foil over a roasting tray will work just fine. Cooking in liquid is the perfect way to develop flavour into the meat. One of my favourite dishes is Slow-cooked Lamb with Anchovies (see recipe page 187) which includes 3 cups of organic bone broth, shallots, garlic, bay leaves, rosemary and thyme. Once the lamb is cooked (5–6 hours) I drain off the liquid and reduce it in a wide frying pan on a high heat – after 10 minutes it becomes a deliciously flavourful and rich jus to serve with the lamb.

Allowing meat protein – whether a steak, a cheek, a fish or a chicken breast – to 'rest' is an important part of cooking it. A steak is a portion of muscle and is home to thousands of neatly aligned muscle fibres that contract when exposed to extreme temperatures. Resting the steak permits the fibres to return to their resting length. It also allows the moisture in the meat to disperse through the entire steak. The end result will be a consistently moist and tender piece of steak. The key to succulent protein is to know what cut you're dealing with and the optimum cooking method, temperature and time.

When it comes to fish and heat, similar rules apply, in that not all fish respond to cooking in the same way. It really comes down to knowing the particular species. For instance, I would cook a piece of salmon (skin on) over a high heat but cook a flathead or whiting fillet at a lower temperature. Fish with greater fat content can tolerate higher temperatures, but the shape and thickness of the fish/fillet needs to be taken into consideration. A thin fish will require a shorter cook time than the thicker fish. And just like meat, fish need to rest, too. The total cook time should include the rest time also. You can refine this with practice, but it's best to pull your fish off the heat just as it nears perfection – the residual heat will finish cooking the fish during the resting period.

The one thing to avoid when cooking meat or fish is to have the heat too low. High heat seals the meat and locks in the moisture. This is called browning or sealing. When the pan heat is too low, the sealing or browning of the meat doesn't occur and so the moisture contained within the protein seeps out and the meat continues to cook in its own juices – otherwise known as stewing. This isn't going to encourage anyone back to your dinner table anytime soon. The browning or sealing phase not only traps the moisture within the protein but also caramelises the outside of the meat to give it texture and flavour. If you've ever thrown your steak on the barbecue prematurely, you'll know what I mean by stewing. It'll cook, yes, but won't have the beautiful caramelisation and flavour of a steak that's thrown on when the temperature is hot. For best results, crank the barbecue 10 minutes before cooking and leave the lid on – it'll get super-hot and burn off any remnants from your previous feast.

How to cook veggies

When it comes to cooking veggies, the same attention to heat applies. Each veggie is different and should be treated so. Also, the type of dish should be taken into consideration. Are the veggies to be added to a piece of protein like a chicken breast, are they to be cooked in broth (as with a soup or stew), or are they to be partially cooked in liquid (as with a stir-fry)? Cooking veggies comes down to their size, type and the desired outcome. Whether you're baking them, steaming them, frying them or boiling them, the most important rule is to not overcook them. Remember, we're trying to entice you and your loved ones to the dinner table time and time again, so presenting flaccid, pale veggies just ain't going to cut it. My mum will hate me for saying this, but despite her being an awesome cook, cooking for the public for nearly 40 years in various pubs in and around London, she never respected the veg. Her stews, pâtés and casseroles were to die for, but she would boil the peas, potatoes and carrots to within an inch of their life and dish them up alongside a magnificent beef and Guinness pie – lucky the pie was so good, I say.

Let's suppose you're roasting some veggies in the oven. Ultimately you want to get some beautiful caramelisation and nuttiness, so it's necessary to take into account the size of the cuts and the type of veg. Cutting all the veg the same size and cooking for the same amount of time will have different results – some veggies will be cooked to perfection, others will be overcooked or undercooked. The same applies for wet dishes like casseroles, stews and curries – the size of the cut and the type of veg will determine the cooking time. One way to avoid poorly cooked veggies is to add them to the oven or pot at different times, placing the 'woodier' veggies (such as potatoes, turnips, swedes and pumpkin) in earlier than veggies such as peas, spinach and cabbage.

Lastly, remember there's always residual heat in the pot, dish or pan, and this residual heat will continue to cook the veggies, so for great results pull them from the heat just before they're perfect and let the residual heat do the rest.

2. HERBS AND SPICES

Herbs are the fresh and dried leaves of plants, such as thyme or mint, and spices are their flowers, fruit, seeds, bark and roots, such as cinnamon and paprika. It is possible for a herb and a spice to originate from the same plant, as is the case with coriander – the seeds, the spice, is generally more pungent than the leaves, the herb.

Herbs and spices sit in our pantry and on the supermarket shelves, where it's easy to take them for granted, but they have had a long history of use for medicinal and flavour purposes, and for preservation to increase the shelf-life of produce. For 40,000–60,000 years, Indigenous Australians have employed herbs, plants and spices, such as wattle seed, sea parsley, salt bush, river mint, native thyme, mountain pepper and lemon myrtle, to enhance the flavour of their food or for medicinal purposes. There is much to learn from this heritage.

In the past, herbs were only available during the warm months of the growing season, and consumers had to suffice with dried herbs at all other times. The business of producing fresh herbs for year-round availability has become one of the fastest-growing agricultural industries.

Adding spices and herbs to food is a cheap and easy way to elevate a dish to a higher level. Using herbs and spices creates nuances, and pairing certain proteins with herbs or a combination of herbs can turn a good dish into a great dish. Some great combinations are:

Lamb and rosemary
Apple and cinnamon
Pork and caraway
Beef and oregano

Chocolate and chilli
Chicken and thyme
Fish and dill

As well as the flavour, herbs and spices carry potent nutritional properties. For example, turmeric activates our BDNF – our brain fertiliser, which promotes the propagation of new neurons (neural biogenesis) and improves the function of existing neurons. In a bid to get smarter, last year I ate turmeric every day, and maybe I did get smarter, but sadly I only looked more stupid with yellow-stained lips and teeth. You win some, you lose some!

Studies have also been conducted to determine whether chilli has any health effects – good or bad. The results seem somewhat inconclusive; however, some increased risk of gastric cancer was noted when high levels of spicy foods were consumed[4] and one study suggests a diet including chilli pepper is linked to a lower mortality rate.[5] With such conflicting findings, just treat chilli as an ingredient that can excite and lift a dish!

3. SALT

Much like spices and herbs, salt has a rich history in connection with the human race. Its original purpose was to preserve food – particularly meat. Salt draws water molecules out of meat or fish and destroys the environment in which the microbes responsible for decay can thrive. It's somewhat hard to imagine these days due to its ubiquity, but salt used to a highly prized commodity. Before the technological efficiencies that followed the industrial revolution, the cost of sourcing and distribution was high, and because the demand for salt was high, it was very expensive. Salt production and trade was a massive economy, with many roads built just to transport salt from place to place, and the effects linger today – for example, the word 'salary' stems from the Latin, meaning a Roman soldier's allowance to buy salt.[6]

Many moons ago I was on a popular reality cooking show in Australia. As I progressed through the show, I learnt the importance of seasoning food throughout the cooking process rather than simply adding salt to a dish once plated. I was repeatedly told by the judges to add more salt. I finally got the message, and by the semi-final was adding so much salt to my cooking that an overly salted swordfish dish saw me exiting the competition. So, yes, you can over-season your food, but there's no excuse for under-seasoning.

Salt brings out the best in a variety of foods. Invest in some good-quality sea salt or Himalayan pink salt and sit it on your kitchen bench for easy and regular access. Table salt is usually heavily refined and mixed with anti-caking agents to prevent clumping so be selective with the salt you use. Table salt is usually iodised, but pink salt naturally has iodine – albeit not in the quantities of iodised salt. The reason that most table salt is iodised is to combat the worldwide issue of iodine deficiencies. Iodine is an essential mineral needed for optimal thyroid function and brain development. A balanced diet will provide enough iodine, which can be found in seaweed, kelp, oysters, prawns and eggs, but if none of those rock your world, a multivitamin will do the trick.

Obviously too much of anything can be detrimental to health, including salt. The Australian National Health and Medical Research Council recommends that adults should consume about 2000 mg of salt, or approximately 1 teaspoon of regular table salt, per day.[7]

¼ teaspoon salt = 575 mg sodium

½ teaspoon salt = 1150 mg sodium

¾ teaspoon salt = 1725 mg sodium

1 teaspoon salt = 2300 mg sodium

Salt as a health food is hugely debated. Studies indicate that there are negative health outcomes from both a low-sodium diet and a high-sodium diet. If consumed in moderation, salt offers many benefits: sodium is crucial for maintaining our bodies' fluid balance, transporting oxygen and nutrients, and supporting the nervous system. Furthermore, if adding some salt to your veggies helps to get them over the line with the family at dinnertime, that's a big win in my book. Life is better with salt . . . and take that with a pinch of salt!

4. LEMON

The humble lemon, aka *Citrus limon*, was introduced to Europeans from Arabia, China and India around the eleventh century. When the Spanish, Dutch and British were sending fleets of ships to discover new territories during the fifteenth century, the seamen lived in unsanitary conditions and with terrible nutrition for long periods of time, resulting in many diseases. One of the most prominent was scurvy. According to James Lind – a Scottish doctor – more British seamen died due to scurvy than to combat with the Spanish and French during this time.[8] Scurvy is brought on by severe and chronic vitamin C deficiency. It manifests in fatigue, loss of appetite, diarrhoea and fever, and can escalate to bleeding gums, loose teeth, bulging eyes and poor bone strength.

In 1740 Lind conducted one of the first recorded clinical trials, giving sailors supplements, which cemented his theory that citrus fruit cured scurvy. This had a huge impact on the health of many seamen in the years to come, and when James Cook sailed for the first time, he took with him syrup of lemon and oranges.

With the availability of fresh produce and supplements, scurvy is less prevalent today, but it may surprise you to learn that it hasn't disappeared altogether, and it can still be cured by lemons.

Lemons are rich in vitamin C. Vitamin C is important in the diet for a number of reasons, including as an antioxidant; in collagen formation, to strengthen skin, blood and bones; to help iron absorption, particularly non-heme iron found in plant-based foods; and in fighting off infections by boosting the immune system, particularly lymphocyte cells.

From a foodie point of view, adding lemon to fish, beef, lamb or vegetables is a cheap and easy way to elevate the dish. This technique works incredibly well with fatty proteins such as salmon or lamb shoulder. Lemon juice can also be incorporated into a salsa or dressing.

5. FERMENTATION

Food fermentation is one of the oldest known uses of biotechnology. Its purpose is to extend the life of fresh produce. Fermented foods have been around longer than hipsters and farmers' markets. Before the rise of multi-flavoured kombucha as all the rage, foods were preserved through naturally occurring fermentation. This process enhances the flavour of the food as well as extending its shelf-life. Nowadays, large-scale production of fermented foods is common, with defined systems of starter cultures used to ensure consistency as well as quality.[9]

Consuming microbes cultivated through fermentation – aka probiotics – is now the buzz and is key to fostering a healthy and robust gut microbiome. The health of our gut plays a significant role in our wellbeing, and fermented foods can help restore the balance. The lack of nutritional diversity in the Western diet can have negative impacts on your gut health. Eating predominantly processed foods, including wheat and sugar, can create a vicious cycle that keeps you craving sweet foods.

But fermented foods and beverages contain healthy bacteria that aids in digestion, assists your body to absorb nutrients and vitamins, supports your immune system and helps to reduce sweet cravings. Once again, an ancient culinary process serves us today from a health perspective as well as a culinary one.

Fermented foods and drinks include yoghurt, pickles, sauerkraut, kimchi, kefir, beers, wines and mead. These can be an acquired taste, but not all healthy things taste good (isn't that right, kale?!). Treat fermented foods as a condiment to your dish. I often add a large tablespoon of kimchi or sauerkraut to my breakfast; it doesn't overpower the hero elements but offers a contrasting sourness to the plate. Given a chance, you might grow to like it.

THE MASTER PLAN

We are living a high-tech existence in an age of ultra-convenience. This way of thinking can spill over into people wanting to get healthy instantaneously. I'm sure we all know someone (or maybe it's you) who is constantly searching for the fast solution to weight management or good health. They'll bunny-hop from one diet trend to another, ultimately never quenching their desire. That's because there *is* no quick fix. Sure, there are strategies for rapid weight loss to help squeeze into the dream wedding dress, but those strategies are not sustainable. So rather than trying to get healthy by the end of your lunchbreak or week, develop a master plan. Your health is determined by what you do most of the time over the greatest period of time, and depending what your starting age is, maybe that will be the next 20, 30, 40 or 60 years.

An integral part of creating a successful master plan is to adjust the lens through which you view health. Some of us perceive health through weight management, good skin, good hair, performance on the athletics field, but if we narrow the focus and look at the smallest moving part in this equation, it'll serve us well. Rather than seeking external markers, let us view health at a cellular level. If our cells are functioning well, all those other things will naturally fall into place.

Once you're looking at cellular health, the focus is then on providing your body with appropriate and adequate inputs for health. In doing this you soon realise that the Western diet is way off track in providing humans with what they require for cellular health.

My focus is on cellular health – specifically, on mitochondrial health – and this focus helps to strip away the fuss, the trends and the buzz words from conversations around what constitutes healthy eating. For me, it's binary in its simplicity. I ask myself, will that food amplify cellular health? Will that drink amplify cellular health? Will that action amplify cellular health? If the answer is yes, then I'll consume it, or if the answer is no, I'll avoid it.

Imagine buying a beautiful plant from the garden centre down the road. You bring it home and it takes pride of place in the lounge room. You neglect it for a number of weeks until brown spots appear on its leaves. To remedy this, you wipe the damaged leaves clean of dust. However, no amount of wiping and dusting of the leaves will rid them of brown spots. You're attempting to find a topical solution for a problem which has its roots elsewhere (pun intended). If the plant was moved to a sunnier spot, given good soil and watered adequately, you'd be giving the plant's cells the right inputs to thrive.

Give the cells what they need and the rest will take care of itself – it's a useful way to view health.

IT'S ALL IN THE TITLE

The key to *any* health plan is to create a framework that is achievable and practical, to ensure adherence over time. Remember, our health will be determined by what we do over the greatest period of time. Therefore it's imperative that we make the relevant changes to improve our lifestyle slowly. So let's lay the foundation and start sculpting our healthy lifestyle. Some of us might have to wean ourselves off sugar, alcohol or medications – this takes time. Some of us might have to learn to cook – this takes time. Some of us might have to address psychological barriers to living a healthy lifestyle, like self-sabotage mechanisms or low self-esteem – this also takes time.

The title of this book refers to a diet that is sustainable for human health *and* for the planet, but to translate that into an individualised health plan that you can subscribe to today, tomorrow, next week and next year, the plan has to be shaped around your daily rituals, habits, preferences, work life, family life and non-negotiables.

Key Takeaways

1. Nutrient-dense foods are 'live foods' (real food) as opposed to manufactured and processed options. Stock your fridge and pantry with plenty of 'live foods', such as well-sourced proteins and veggies.

2. In order to ascend towards a health epidemic, we need to get excited about cooking with real food in our kitchens. Once we are eating a large proportion of our daily intake from our own kitchen, we will not have to rely so heavily on convenient, processed and packaged foods.

3. There are some really simple tips and tricks to help your kitchen creations taste delicious, including seasoning and cooking techniques. Being persistent, diligent and creative with real food in the kitchen will serve you – and your loved ones – well.

Chapter seven

Conclusion

The aim of this book was to discuss the possibility of a sustainable diet – one that fostered human health and environmental harmony. I sought to unpack the current intensive food systems and shine a light on the regenerative alternatives. If we value human health and ecological health, there is a need to look for an alternative approach to the current food system. In a race to systemise, mechanise and industrialise farming, we disconnected with the very plants and animals being farmed . . . along the way, they became just commodities. The value placed on tracing our food back to the farmer, or growing it ourselves, is the key to lifting us into a *good*-health epidemic.

Creating a new, healthy approach to nutrition after following the typical American diet for decades comes with a bucketload of challenges. But common sense seems to be prevailing, with more and more people choosing to adopt a natural diet. By that I don't necessarily mean a diet of zebra, lizards and insects, but a diet free of refined and processed foods. It just makes sense to give our bodies what they have been designed over millennia to function on.

For human health to be optimal, we need to endorse a real-food diet. This is perhaps nothing new to most of us, but there is another layer to all this, and that's *where* that natural food has come from. Nutritional health is at its peak with naturally sourced food, from ethical sources. If you make your food decisions based on this food system, you'll also be supporting greater animal welfare and ecological health. Science has pushed us in the direction of gut health within the last decade, highlighting the importance of fostering a rich, diverse and robust ecosystem within our colon. The implications for health are huge and should be informing decisions around food, nutrition and lifestyle.

I'm sure you're familiar with the adage 'we are what we eat'. It makes absolute sense, right? Author Michael Pollan expanded on this with 'we are what what we eat eats, too'[1] – an accurate assessment of the fact that we inherit the foods consumed by the animals or plants we eat. All the more reason to support natural food systems!

Regenerative farming poses challenges – most definitely it is at the mercy of climate, weather and natural forces – but it's a sustainable approach which resonates with our DNA. It's in our genetic blueprint to work with nature to harvest food; we did it for 2.5 million years. As my farmer friend Mick explains, farming is about working with nature, not against it, and allowing the principle of farming to mimic nature.

Responsible and ethical farming leads to human and ecological health. Ethical animal husbandry and crops grown in sympathy with nature is the solution; only when dealing with a food system that supports animal welfare, ecology and human health are we able to make an honest and objective appraisal of what we eat for personal health. To me, this is the ultimate scenario: our dietary preference supported by ethical produce, irrespective of whether we eat meat or not. We need access to good-quality food – food that is devoid of harmful pesticides, fertilisers, antibiotics and hormones.

With the growth of interest in food sovereignty, I believe we have seen the worst of industrialised farming. Public pressure will continue to influence decisions made by farmers and producers, ultimately steering us in more ethical directions. Farmers unable or unwilling to adapt to the pressure could face a downturn in sales. This is how change happens; new thoughts and ideologies brew and fester until a critical mass is reached. It's at this point that the persuasive power is tangible.

We are all part of nature, but for the last 100 years we have not served our planet positively. We have held an imperialistic view of the world; we have abused our rights, blinkered to the consequences of our behaviours. Those behaviours and actions are being felt now with global warming, environmental degradation and disease epidemics. Engaging in and supporting a sustainable diet is the way to begin to unwind the damage done. Eating fresh, ethical produce is paramount to our health and the health of the planet.

I look forward to seeing the direction we take over the next 100 years.

THE CUTE CAT STORY

The nightly TV news tends to sign off with a cute story to leave you feeling good about the world. Well, here's my version of the cute cat story . . .

If you had to pick which country is leading the charge with sustainable farming as an attempt to lessen the harm done to the environment, Bolivia probably wouldn't be the first on your list. However, the government of Bolivia has recently invested

$40 million to support small- and medium-scale farmers in food production. Marisol Solano, Deputy Minister of Rural Development and Agriculture, stated that more than twenty food security projects are already underway across the country, with financial support being given to breeding livestock and farming fish, as well as increasing the production of crops like potatoes, tomatoes, wheat, vegetables, coffee and cocoa. By enhancing and supporting local production, Bolivia aims to become entirely self-sufficient by 2020. Bravo Bolivia!

Since 2014 they've witnessed a 25 per cent increase in food production, and with the aim being to sustain this growth rate for the coming year, it seems the country is not too far off from achieving its ambitions. Reducing or halting imports would not only help improve the livelihoods of local farmers and businesses, it would also cut down on emissions while addressing overarching global issues like unemployment, hunger and poverty.

This is a huge step in the right direction for sustainable farming. Hopefully the Bolivian example can inspire other countries to follow suit.

Your body deserves the best inputs you can provide. Tracing your ingredients back to ethical sources will do much for your health, and the planet's.

Be healthy, be happy.

PART TWO

Recipes for a sustainable diet

A note on ingredients

Your nutrition has the biggest impact on general health. The path to optimal health is to ensure a broad and diverse array of fresh and unprocessed foods, including ethically raised animal produce (if you choose to eat meat, that is) and plenty of aboveground vegetables.

Wherever possible, source good-quality produce including organic veggies, eggs, chicken and meat, as well as sustainable seafood. It's not easy or practical to achieve this 100 per cent of the time but taking steps towards this is preferable for your health, animal welfare and the state of the planet.

I have some non-negotiables when shopping, which include only grass-fed/-finished meat, organic eggs (or biodynamic) and organic chicken. When I have the budget and access to organic vegetables, I'll use them, but that's not always the case so I make do with supermarket veg. Even if organic/grass-fed produce is out of reach financially or literally, then stocking your fridge and pantry with fresh, whole and unprocessed food will still move the needle of your health and the health of your family.

Introduction to recipes

So far we have discussed the theoretical side of a sustainable diet, or the *why*. Now is the exciting part of the book when we discuss the *how*, and by the how I mean cooking. Part two shares over 100 recipes that I've put together to assist you in living a healthy lifestyle, as well as supporting sustainable or regenerative food systems. With this many recipes there really is something for everyone – so please have a rummage through, as I'm confident there'll be a few that get you salivating. With any recipe, you're welcome (actually encouraged) to simply use mine as a framework and layer in your own preferences. If you want more or less salt, spice, tang, acidity or umami then adjust to your liking.

I have included some recipes and ingredients which some might view as obscure or even controversial – these are deliberate choices and completely in line with the theme of sustainability. We have to think outside the square to reassess our food supply, which is why I've included some 'obscure' foods . . . but don't knock it till you've tried it.

It's vitally important to understand the *why* behind a lifestyle – understanding the mechanics is paramount to success – but the *how* cannot be undervalued. Having the confidence and wherewithal to shop, prep and cook delicious healthy food will be the best way out of the disease epidemic currently faced in the industrialised world. I hope these recipes can help you get excited about being in your kitchen cooking real food with love.

Happy cooking!

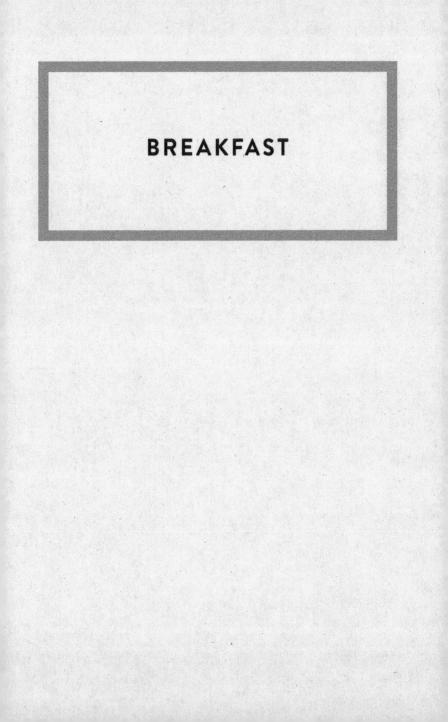

BREAKFAST

Crab Omelette

Ask your friendly fishmonger for some white crabmeat, which is more delicate and sweet than brown.

SERVES 1

3 organic eggs, *lightly whisked*
½ teaspoon chilli flakes
¼ bunch of coriander, *leaves chopped*
100g white crabmeat
1 tablespoon organic ghee
sea salt and freshly ground black pepper, to taste

1. In a mixing bowl, combine the eggs, chilli flakes, coriander and crabmeat. Lightly whisk, then season with salt and pepper.
2. Place a frying pan over a medium heat and add the ghee. Pour the egg mixture into the pan and cook for 2–3 minutes, or until golden on the underside. Gently lift the edge of the omelette, flip over and continue to cook for 1–2 minutes, or until cooked through.
3. Remove from the pan, season again with salt and pepper, and serve.

Omega Bowl

This little bowl of omega goodness is a winner at my restaurants.

SERVES 1

4 tablespoons shredded coconut
2 tablespoons hemp seeds
1 tablespoon walnuts, *crushed*
1 tablespoon pistachios, *crushed*
1 tablespoon hazelnuts, *crushed*
1 tablespoon pumpkin seeds
1 tablespoon sunflower seeds
1 tablespoon flaxseeds
1 tablespoon sesame seeds
small handful of fresh or frozen blueberries
small handful of fresh or frozen blackberries
200g unsweetened coconut yoghurt
1 teaspoon hemp oil
1 teaspoon honey

1. Combine all the dry elements in a mixing bowl (you could make a large batch ahead of time if you wanted to). If using frozen berries, remove from the freezer to thaw for 10 minutes.
2. Combine with the berries, coconut yoghurt, hemp oil and honey, stirring to allow some of the berries to bleed into the yoghurt.

BLT with Black Pudding

SERVES 1

1 tablespoon olive oil
1 gluten-free black sausage, *cut into 1cm discs*
½ avocado
juice of 1 lemon
½ teaspoon chilli flakes
¼ bunch of parsley, *leaves chopped*
2 lettuce leaves
small handful of cherry tomatoes, halved
1 organic egg, *boiled*
1 tablespoon Horseradish Mayo (see recipe page 244)
sea salt and freshly ground black pepper, to taste

1. Heat a small frying pan over a high heat and add 1 teaspoon of the olive oil. Add the black sausage and fry for 2 minutes on each side, or until browned. Remove from the heat and allow to rest.
2. In a mixing bowl, combine the avocado, lemon juice, chilli flakes and parsley and mash together roughly with a fork. Season with salt and pepper.
3. In another bowl, combine the lettuce, cherry tomatoes and remaining olive oil. Season to taste.
4. Serve the avocado mash with the egg, black sausage, the rocket and tomato salad, and Horseradish Mayo.

Bacon and Broccoli Frittata

A frittata is a great meal at any time of the day. It is a perfect dish to adapt to whatever vegetables you have that need using up. You could use squash, asparagus, carrots, beans, or just about anything else.

SERVES 4

200g free-range pancetta or bacon, *chopped*
2 tablespoons organic butter
2 shallots, *peeled and quartered*
1 teaspoon fresh thyme leaves
½ teaspoon chilli flakes
1 bunch of tenderstem broccoli, *trimmed*
6 organic eggs, *lightly whisked*
¼ bunch of parsley, *leaves roughly chopped*
sea salt and freshly ground black pepper, to taste

1. Preheat your oven to 170°C.
2. Place an ovenproof frying pan over a high heat, add the chopped bacon or pancetta and cook until the fat is rendered and the meat is crisp. Remove from the pan and set aside.
3. Wipe the pan, return to a high heat and add 1 tablespoon of the butter. Add the shallots, thyme and chilli flakes and cook for 2–3 minutes. Add the broccoli and cook for 4–5 minutes, or until the broccoli is charred a little. Transfer the contents of the pan to a bowl and set aside.
4. Return the pan to the heat, add the remaining tablespoon of butter, then add the eggs. Scatter the broccoli mixture evenly over the eggs and add the bacon and parsley. Bake in the oven for 8 minutes, or until cooked through.
5. Transfer the frittata to a chopping board, season with salt and pepper, and serve.

Fried Egg Omelette

Breakfast shouldn't be a time to scrimp on veggies. Here's a recipe that packs in a bunch of them to start your day in the right way.

SERVES 1

1 tablespoon coconut oil

1 tablespoon olive oil

1 shallot, *peeled and halved*

1 garlic clove, *sliced*

3 tenderstem broccoli, *trimmed and cut in half lengthways*

1 asparagus spear, *trimmed and cut in half lengthways*

1 tablespoon capers

3 organic eggs

2 tablespoons sauerkraut, to serve

sea salt and freshly ground black pepper, to taste

1. Place a frying pan over a medium heat and add both oils. Add the shallot and garlic and cook for 2–3 minutes.
2. Add the broccoli, asparagus and capers and cook for a further 3–4 minutes, or until the heads of the broccoli begin to char.
3. Reduce the heat to low then crack the eggs in, allowing the egg whites to cover the bottom of the pan. Cook until the eggs are done to your liking.
4. Using a spatula, gently lift one side of the omelette up and across, folding it in half. Season with salt and pepper and serve with sauerkraut.

Shallots, Tomatoes and Eggs

Another breakfast recipe which squeezes in the veggies ...

SERVES 2

1 tablespoon coconut oil
1 tablespoon olive oil
2 shallots, *peeled and halved*
4 garlic cloves, *sliced*
2 tomatoes, *quartered*
4 organic eggs
sea salt and freshly ground black pepper, to taste

1. Place a frying pan over a low–medium heat and add both oils. Add the shallots and garlic and cook for 3–4 minutes, stirring occasionally.
2. Turn the heat to medium and cook the tomatoes for 2–3 minutes.
3. Turn the heat to low and crack in the eggs. Cook until the eggs are done to your liking.
4. Remove from the heat, season with salt and pepper, and serve.

Pea and Pesto Omelette

If you make a big batch of the pesto ahead of time, you can keep it refrigerated for weeks.

SERVES 1

50g frozen peas
3 organic eggs
1 tablespoon organic butter
1 tablespoon Pesto (see recipe page 241)
3–4 snow pea tendrils
sea salt and freshly ground black pepper, to taste

1. Place the peas in tepid water for 5 minutes. Drain.
2. In a bowl, gently whisk the eggs and season with salt and pepper. Set aside.
3. Place a frying pan over a medium heat and add the butter. Once the butter begins to foam, add the eggs and scatter over the peas. Cook for 3–4 minutes, or until cooked to your liking.
4. Dot the pesto on top, add the snow pea tendrils, season with more salt and pepper, and fold over. Serve.

Scrambled Eggs with Pesto

Take your scrambled eggs to the next level with the addition of my delicious pesto.

SERVES 1

1 teaspoon organic butter or ghee
3 organic eggs
1 tablespoon Pesto (see recipe page 241)
sea salt and freshly ground black pepper, to taste

1. Place a frying pan over a low heat and add the butter or ghee.
2. In a bowl, lightly whisk the eggs and season with salt and pepper. Pour into the pan and, using a wooden spoon, gently stir.
3. Continue to cook until almost done to your liking. With 30 seconds of cooking time remaining, add the pesto and stir through. Remove from the heat, season again with salt and pepper, if desired, and serve.

Pea and Pancetta Omelette

A simple breakfast or lunch item which is best when good-quality ingredients are sourced.

SERVES 4

150g frozen peas
150g free-range pancetta or bacon, *roughly chopped*
12 organic eggs, *lightly whisked*
1 tablespoon organic butter
¼ bunch of parsley, *leaves chopped*
¼ bunch of chives, *chopped*
sea salt and freshly ground black pepper, to taste

1. Place the peas in a bowl of tepid water.
2. Place a large frying pan over a high heat and add the chopped pancetta or bacon. Cook, stirring, until the fat is rendered and the meat is crisp. Remove from the pan and set aside.
3. Season the eggs with salt and pepper. Drain the peas.
4. Return the frying pan to a medium heat and add the butter. Pour in the eggs, add the pancetta and peas and cook for 3–4 minutes, or until the underside of the omelette is cooked.
5. Scatter the chopped herbs over one side of the omelette and flip the opposite side over. Continue to cook until done to your liking. Season and serve.

Green Bowl with Cashew Cheese and Coconut Mint Dressing

SERVES 1

40g steamed peas
40g steamed green beans
4–5 steamed asparagus spears
handful of baby spinach leaves
2 kale leaves, *finely chopped*
3–4 tablespoons Coconut Mint Dressing (see recipe page 245)
2 tablespoons lemon juice
¼ bunch of mint, *leaves picked*
¼ bunch of parsley, *leaves picked*
1 tablespoon micro herbs
1 tablespoon Cashew Cheese (see recipe page 242)
sea salt and freshly ground black pepper, to taste

1. In a large mixing bowl, combine the peas, beans, asparagus, baby spinach and kale. Apply the Coconut Mint Dressing, then add the lemon juice, mint, parsley and micro herbs. Toss to combine.
2. Season with salt and pepper, and serve the salad with Cashew Cheese.

BRT

A twist on the classic BLT, with rocket and parsley.

SERVES 1

3 free-range bacon rashers
½ avocado
juice of 1 lemon
½ teaspoon chilli flakes
¼ bunch of parsley, *leaves chopped*
small handful of rocket
small handful of cherry tomatoes, halved
1 tablespoon olive oil
1 organic egg, *boiled or fried*
1 tablespoon Horseradish Mayo (see recipe page 244)
sea salt and freshly ground black pepper, to taste

1. Place a small frying pan over a high heat and add the bacon. Fry until cooked to your liking.
2. Meanwhile, in a mixing bowl combine the avocado, lemon juice, chilli flakes and parsley, and mash together roughly with a fork. Season with salt and pepper.
3. In another bowl, combine the rocket, cherry tomatoes and olive oil. Season to taste.
4. Serve the avocado mash with the bacon, egg, rocket and tomato salad, and Horseradish Mayo.

Gooding Smash

This is a little 'treaty' without the 'guilty'.

SERVES 1

handful of frozen berries of your choice
4 tablespoons coconut cream or unsweetened coconut yoghurt
1 tablespoon peanut butter
1 tablespoon hemp seeds
1 tablespoon hemp oil
1 teaspoon honey (optional)
1 teaspoon cacao nibs

1. Place all the ingredients in a serving bowl and give it a little swirl or two.
2. Let rest for 10–15 minutes for the berries to thaw, then serve.

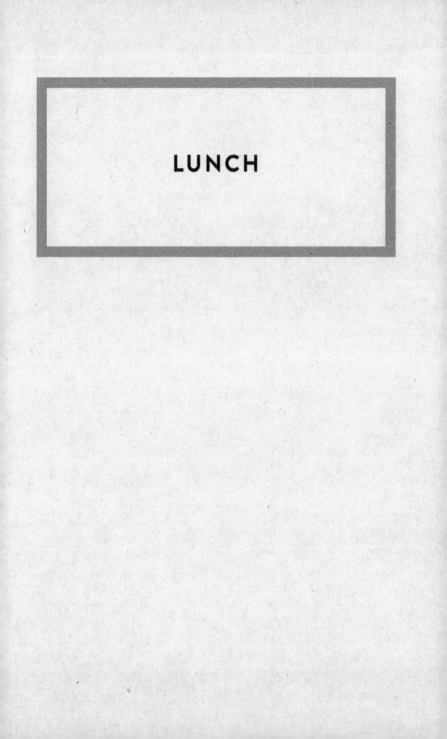

LUNCH

Tomato Salad

This is a wonderfully simple salad, and a recipe that allows the ingredients to speak for themselves.

SERVES 2

8–10 heirloom tomatoes, *roughly chopped*
2 celery stalks, *trimmed and chopped*
1 small red onion, *sliced*
1 garlic clove, *grated*
½ bunch of basil, *leaves torn*
1 bunch of parsley, *leaves and stalks chopped*
3 tablespoons baby capers
1 tablespoon lemon juice
1 tablespoon red wine vinegar
4 tablespoons olive oil
sea salt and freshly ground black pepper, to taste

1. Combine all the ingredients in a large mixing bowl. Leave for 5 minutes for the flavours to combine.
2. Adjust the seasonings and mix again prior to serving.

Chopped Salad

In my house, this type of salad is usually on the table a day or so before the next big food shop. I rummage around in the fridge and pantry and try to use up any veggies that are getting close to their use-by date.

SERVES 2

3 tablespoons capers
1 cucumber, *chopped*
½ bunch of parsley, *leaves picked*
½ head of broccoli, *cut into florets*
1 celery stalk, *chopped*
handful of snow peas, *trimmed*
3 tomatoes, *chopped*
handful of pistachios
large handful of baby spinach leaves
sea salt and freshly ground black pepper, to taste

DRESSING

1 teaspoon Dijon mustard
3 tablespoons olive oil
1 tablespoon lemon juice
pinch of salt
pinch of black pepper

1. Combine the ingredients for the dressing in a small jar, cover and shake vigorously. Set aside.
2. Combine all the salad ingredients in a large mixing bowl and gently toss. Add the dressing and toss again. Add more olive oil or dressing if desired. Season again with salt and pepper, and serve.

Chargrilled Asparagus with Egg

This is a great light lunch option. It's also good as a side to a
fish or chicken dish.

SERVES 2

2 tablespoons olive oil
16–20 asparagus spears, *trimmed*
juice of ½ lemon
½ teaspoon chilli flakes
¼ bunch of tarragon, *leaves chopped*
¼ bunch of dill, *leaves chopped*
2–3 tablespoons Tahini Dressing with Capers (see recipe page 252)
4 organic eggs, *boiled*
sea salt and freshly ground black pepper, to taste

1. Heat a griddle pan over a high heat (or heat your barbecue to high)
   and add 1 tablespoon of the olive oil. Add the asparagus and cook,
   rotating every 30 seconds, until charred. Remove from the heat.
2. Place the asparagus in a large mixing bowl and add the lemon juice,
   chilli flakes, tarragon, dill and the remaining olive oil. Toss.
3. Transfer to a serving bowl/dish, add the tahini dressing and season
   with salt and pepper. Serve with the eggs.

Kebabs with Coconut Yoghurt

Okay, okay, I know I've included more than a few recipes influenced by my trip to the Middle East, but it's hard to not get inspired by travel to foreign countries. After five days surrounded by the opulence of Dubai, I craved basic street food and was recommended a kebab restaurant that hadn't changed for 70 years. With only one item on the menu, it was a good thing it was delicious!

SERVES 4

2 garlic cloves
½ teaspoon grated lemon zest
1 teaspoon dried or fresh thyme
1 tablespoon dried or fresh oregano
2 tablespoons olive oil
4 organic lamb steaks, *chopped into 3–4cm chunks*
1 tablespoon lemon juice
400g unsweetened coconut yoghurt
¼ bunch of parsley, *leaves roughly chopped*
2 red peppers, *roughly chopped*
1 lemon, for squeezing
olive oil, for drizzling
4 heirloom tomatoes, *chopped*
sea salt and freshly ground black pepper, to taste

1. Soak 8 wooden skewers in a bowl of water for 10 minutes.
2. In a mortar and pestle, pound the garlic cloves with the lemon zest, thyme and oregano. Transfer to a bowl, add the olive oil and season with salt and pepper.
3. Add the chopped lamb, mixing well to coat. Set aside for 30 minutes to marinate.
4. In separate bowl, combine the lemon juice, coconut yoghurt and parsley. Season with salt and pepper.
5. Heat your barbecue to high or place a frying pan over a high heat.
6. Thread the lamb and pepper pieces alternately onto the skewers. Barbecue or fry, turning often, for 15 minutes, or until cooked through. Remove from the heat and allow to rest.
7. Squeeze some lemon juice over the lamb and season again with salt and pepper. Drizzle olive oil over the tomatoes and serve with the lamb skewers and the yoghurt sauce.

Hilton Niçoise with Roasted New Potatoes

Staying at the Hilton Sharjah during my visit to the United Arab Emirates, I discovered this beautiful yet classic niçoise salad. They used a very acidic dressing – right up my alley.

SERVES 4

16 new potatoes
5 tablespoons olive oil
400g MSC tuna steak
1 cos lettuce, *chopped*
large handful of chopped chicory
1 red onion, *chopped*
4 organic eggs, *boiled and halved*
¼ bunch of dill, *chopped*
sea salt and freshly ground black pepper, to taste

DRESSING

1 teaspoon seeded mustard
1 tablespoon red wine vinegar
3 tablespoons olive oil

1. Preheat your oven to 220°C.
2. Cook the potatoes in boiling salted water for 10 minutes.
3. Pour 4 tablespoons of olive oil into a baking tray. Add the potatoes and roast for 40 minutes, or until the potato skins are crisp. Remove from the oven, sprinkle with salt and pepper and allow to cool.
4. Place a frying pan over a high heat and add the remaining tablespoon of olive oil. When very hot, add the tuna and sear on both sides for 30 seconds (times will vary according to thickness of the fish). Remove from the heat.
5. In a bowl, combine the cos lettuce, chicory, red onion, eggs and potatoes.
6. Make the dressing by whisking together the mustard, red wine vinegar and olive oil. Pour on the salad and gently toss.
7. Slice the tuna and add to the salad, sprinkle with dill, season with salt and pepper, and serve.

Chicken Skewers

SERVES 4

200g unsweetened coconut yoghurt

1 tablespoon garam masala

1 teaspoon curry powder

1 tablespoon coconut oil

8–10 organic chicken thigh fillets

1 small punnet of cherry tomatoes, *halved*

1 Lebanese cucumber, *sliced*

1 red onion, *sliced*

¼ bunch of coriander, *leaves chopped*

1 long green chilli, *sliced*

2 tablespoons lemon juice

sea salt and freshly ground black pepper, to taste

1. Soak 12–15 wooden skewers in a bowl of water for 10 minutes.

2. In a mixing bowl, combine the coconut yoghurt, garam masala, curry powder and coconut oil. Season to taste with salt.

3. Line up 2 chicken fillets next to each other and thread three parallel skewers through both thighs. Now cut through the thighs either side of the middle skewer to create three separate skewers. Repeat with the remaining chicken thighs.

4. Coat the chicken skewers in the coconut and spice marinade and leave, covered, for 20 minutes.

5. Preheat your oven grill to high.

6. Place the chicken skewers on a baking tray and cook under the grill for 10 minutes. Turn the skewers and continue to cook for 8–10 minutes, or until cooked through. Remove from the oven and leave to rest for 3–5 minutes.

7. Combine the cherry tomatoes, cucumber, onion, coriander, chilli and lemon juice in a bowl. Gently toss. Season the salad and serve with the chicken skewers.

Pan-fried Hake with Caper Butter

I was fortunate enough to demonstrate this great recipe while presenting at the Sharjah International Book Fair (United Arab Emirates) early in 2019.

SERVES 2

75g organic butter
3 garlic cloves, *minced*
2 tablespoons capers
juice and grated zest of 1 lemon
4 tablespoons chopped dill
2 hake fillets
sea salt and freshly ground black pepper, to taste

1. Place a small saucepan over a low heat and add the butter, garlic, capers and lemon zest. Cook for 10 minutes, then add the dill and lemon juice and continue to cook for 5 minutes.
2. Place a frying pan over a high heat and add 4–5 tablespoons of the butter mixture to the pan. Add the fish and cook for 2–3 minutes on each side (time will vary according to the thickness of the fish).
3. Remove from the heat, season with salt and pepper, and serve with any remaining caper butter drizzled over.

Roasted Butternut Salad

Fresh and light, not to mention deliciously healthy – perfection!

SERVES 4

½ butternut squash, *peeled and chopped into 2–3cm pieces*
1 large sweet potato, *peeled and chopped into 2–3cm pieces*
2 tablespoons Moroccan seasoning
3–4 tablespoons olive oil
1 large carrot, *grated*
1 large courgette, *cut into ribbons or julienned*
1 red onion, *sliced*
1 small punnet of cherry tomatoes, *halved*
½ bunch of coriander, *leaves chopped*
½ bunch of mint, *leaves chopped*
juice and grated zest of 1 lemon
4 tablespoons toasted flaked almonds
250ml Coconut Mint Dressing (see recipe page 245)
sea salt and freshly ground black pepper, to taste

1. Preheat your oven to 190°C.
2. In a large mixing bowl, combine the squash, sweet potato, Moroccan seasoning and oil. Tip into a baking tray and roast for 40 minutes, or until the vegetables are softened and browned. Remove from the oven and allow to cool.
3. In another large mixing bowl, combine all the remaining ingredients except the dressing. Add the roasted vegetables and gently toss.
4. Season with salt and pepper and serve with the Coconut Mint Dressing.

Kelp Noodles with Pesto

Kelp is so incredibly easy to prepare and is low in calories. Kelp noodles – available from most health food stores or online – are a great low-carb substitute for pasta or rice.

SERVES 2

500g kelp noodles
1 teaspoon salt
juice of 1 lemon
2–3 tablespoons Pesto (see recipe page 241)
¼ bunch of coriander, *leaves chopped*
¼ bunch of mint, *leaves chopped*
4 tablespoons crushed raw cashews
1 tablespoon chilli oil
1 punnet of cherry tomatoes, *halved*
sea salt and freshly ground black pepper, to taste

1. Place the kelp noodles in a large bowl and cover with warm water. Add the salt and lemon juice and leave to soak for 1 hour.
2. Drain the noodles and combine with the pesto. Gently stir in the chopped coriander and mint.
3. Transfer to a serving plate, sprinkle with crushed cashews and drizzle with 1 teaspoon of chilli oil. Add the cherry tomatoes and drizzle with the remaining chilli oil.
4. Season to taste with salt and pepper, and serve.

Mexican Tuna with Grapefruit, Avocado and Fennel

This is a light and refreshing recipe, perfect for a summer's lunch.

SERVES 4

500g MSC tuna steak, *cut into 2cm chunks*
2 avocados, *diced*
2 baby fennel bulbs, *trimmed and thinly sliced*
½ red onion, *thinly sliced*
½ bunch of coriander, *leaves picked*
1 ruby grapefruit, *segmented and roughly chopped*
2 tablespoons pickled jalapeños
2 heirloom tomatoes, *chopped*

DRESSING

4 tablespoons olive oil
2 tablespoons lime juice
1 garlic clove, *crushed*
½ teaspoon ground chipotle
sea salt and freshly ground black pepper, to taste

1. Combine the ingredients for the dressing in a small jar, cover and shake vigorously. Set aside.
2. In a large mixing bowl, combine all the remaining ingredients and gently toss. Add the dressing and toss once again.
3. Adjust seasonings and serve.

Prawn Cocktail Salad with Coriander Mayo

Growing up in my mum and dad's pubs, prawn cocktail with marie rose sauce was one of the fancier starters on the menu – something we offered only on special occasions. Thirty years on, it's still a great dish.

SERVES 4

4 tablespoons olive oil

zest of 2 lemons, *grated*

4 garlic cloves, *crushed*

2–3 long red chillies, *finely chopped*

½ bunch of coriander, *leaves picked, stalks finely chopped*

28 MSC cooked peeled prawns

2 avocados, *sliced*

2 baby cos lettuces, *leaves roughly chopped*

1 punnet of medley cherry tomatoes, *halved*

1 tablespoon macadamia oil

2–3 tablespoons lemon juice

4–6 tablespoons Coriander Mayo (see recipe page 243)

sea salt and freshly ground black pepper, to taste

1. In a large mixing bowl, combine the olive oil, lemon zest, garlic, chillies and coriander stalks. Stir well before adding the prawns. Toss to ensure the prawns are coated in the oil, then pop in the fridge for 30 minutes.

2. In a mixing bowl, combine the avocados, cos lettuces, cherry tomatoes and coriander leaves.

3. Add the prawns to the salad. Drizzle with macadamia oil and lemon juice, and season with salt and pepper. Serve with Coriander Mayo.

Surf and Turf with Horseradish Mayo

Much like the prawn cocktail, this dish is a throwback to the '70s and '80s. It's still delicious.

SERVES 2

2 grass-fed/-finished rump steaks

50g organic butter, plus 1 teaspoon, extra

1–2 garlic cloves, *crushed*

1 bunch of tenderstem broccoli, *trimmed*

1 bunch of asparagus, *trimmed*

juice of 1 lemon

4–6 MSC cooked peeled prawns

2 tablespoons olive oil

2–4 tablespoons Horseradish Mayo (see recipe page 244)

sea salt and freshly ground black pepper, to taste

1. Remove the steaks from the fridge 30 minutes prior to cooking. Season both sides with salt and pepper.
2. Combine the 50g of butter and the garlic in a bowl.
3. Bring a saucepan of salted water to the boil and add the broccoli and asparagus. Cook for 4–5 minutes.
4. Meanwhile, place a frying pan over a high heat. Put half the butter and garlic mixture into the pan and place both steaks in. Cook for 3–4 minutes on each side (or to your preference) before removing from the pan and placing on a chopping board to rest. (Don't wash the pan.)
5. Drain the veggies, add half the lemon juice and the 1 teaspoon of butter, and toss to coat. Set aside.
6. Meanwhile, add the remaining garlic butter to the hot steak pan and throw in the prawns for a few minutes, or until warmed through. Remove from the heat, drizzle with the remaining lemon juice, and season with salt and pepper.
7. Serve with the veggies and some Horseradish Mayo.

Chicken and Fennel Soup

SERVES 6

2 tablespoons organic butter
1 onion, *chopped*
4 garlic cloves, *chopped*
6 shallots, *trimmed and chopped*
2 carrots, *sliced*
2 fennel bulbs, *trimmed and quartered*
½ bunch of rosemary
1 teaspoon dried sage
1 organic chicken
1 bunch of asparagus, *trimmed and chopped*
½ bunch of parsley, *leaves chopped*
sea salt and freshly ground black pepper, to taste

1. Place a large saucepan over a medium heat and add the butter. Add the onion, garlic, shallots, carrots and fennel and sauté for 3–4 minutes. Add the rosemary and sage and cook, stirring, for 1–2 minutes.
2. Place the whole chicken in the pot, cover with water and season with salt and pepper. Bring to the boil, reduce the heat to low and simmer for 1½ hours, or until the chicken is cooked through. Pop the asparagus in the pot 10 minutes before the end of cooking time.
3. Remove the saucepan from the heat, extract the chicken and place on a chopping board. Strip the meat from the carcass and return to the broth, together with the parsley. Add salt and pepper to taste.

Mouth-watering Baked Salmon

I'm not the type of cook who claims to have a signature dish, but I do know that this often gets a run-out. The exact recipe is always changing slightly but the roots stay the same.

SERVES 4

150g unsweetened coconut yoghurt
1 long red chilli, *chopped*
1 teaspoon sumac
juice and grated zest of 1 lemon, plus 1 tablespoon juice, extra
1 tablespoon tahini
800g skinless MSC salmon fillets, *pin-boned*
¼ bunch of coriander, *chopped*
¼ bunch of parsley, *chopped*
handful of pistachios, *chopped*
sea salt and freshly ground black pepper, to taste

1. Preheat your oven to 180°C.
2. In a large mixing bowl, combine the yoghurt, chilli, sumac, lemon juice and zest, and tahini. Season to taste with salt and pepper. Set aside.
3. Line a baking tray with baking paper and place the salmon fillets on top. Bake for 18–20 minutes, or until cooked to your liking.
4. Meanwhile, in a small bowl, combine the coriander, parsley, pistachios and the extra lemon juice.
5. Remove the salmon from the oven and place on a serving dish. Spoon the yoghurt mixture on top, then sprinkle with the herb mixture. Season and serve.

Butterflied Herbed Chook

It's possible to cook the whole chicken, but butterflying it will speed up the cooking time. Simply use a pair of meat scissors to cut the backbone out, or ask your friendly butcher to do it for you.

SERVES 4

4 tablespoons olive oil
2 teaspoons chopped fresh thyme leaves
1 teaspoon chopped fresh rosemary leaves
1 teaspoon smoked paprika
½ teaspoon sweet paprika
½ teaspoon cayenne pepper
grated zest of 1 lemon
4 garlic cloves, *crushed*
1 organic chicken, *butterflied*
sea salt and freshly ground black pepper, to taste

1. Preheat your oven to 200°C.
2. In a mixing bowl, combine the oil, herbs, spices, lemon zest, garlic and salt and pepper to your taste. Place the chicken in the bowl and toss to ensure it is coated in the spice mixture.
3. Line a baking tray with baking paper. Transfer the chicken to the tray, season with salt and pepper, and roast for 35 minutes, or until cooked through.
4. Allow chicken to rest for 5 minutes before serving.

Raw Green Salad

Apple cider vinegar is available in most supermarkets and health food stores. It is great to use in dressings to add acidity or to take as an elixir for its probiotic benefit.

SERVES 1

2 courgettes, *grated*
large handful of baby spinach leaves
¼ bunch of coriander, *chopped*
¼ bunch of mint, *chopped*
¼ bunch of parsley, *chopped*
1 tablespoon pumpkin seeds
1 tablespoon chopped pistachios

DRESSING

3 tablespoons olive oil
1 tablespoon apple cider vinegar
½ teaspoon chilli flakes
1 teaspoon Dijon mustard
sea salt and freshly ground black pepper, to taste

1. Combine the ingredients for the dressing in a small jar, cover and shake vigorously. Set aside.
2. In a large mixing bowl, combine all the salad ingredients. Gently toss, then add the dressing and toss again. Serve.

Crispy Cod with Sweet Peas

The balance of butter, lemon juice, fleshy fish and sweet peas is hard to beat.

SERVES 4

80g frozen peas
150g green beans, *trimmed*
2 tablespoons olive oil
4 cod fillets, skin on
100g organic butter
2 tablespoons capers
1 garlic clove, *thinly sliced*
¼ bunch of dill, *chopped*
juice of 1 lemon
sea salt and freshly ground black pepper, to taste

1. Bring a small saucepan of salted water to the boil and drop in the peas and beans. Blanch for 1 minute, then drain and dunk into iced water. Drain again and set aside.
2. Place a large frying pan over a high heat and add the olive oil. Season the skin of the fish with salt and pepper and place, skin side down, in the pan. Cook for 6 minutes, or until crisp. Flip and cook for a further 2 minutes, or until cooked through. Remove from the pan and set aside, loosely covered with foil.
3. In the fish pan, heat the butter over a medium heat and add the capers and garlic. Cook until the butter begins to brown – about 4–5 minutes. With 1 minute of cooking time remaining, throw in the peas, beans, dill and lemon juice.
4. Serve the sauce over the fish. Season and serve.

Beef Tartare

My favourite local French restaurant serves this classic dish. It's important to start with good-quality produce, including grass-fed/-finished beef and an organic egg.

SERVES 2

350g grass-fed/-finished sirloin steak
1 teaspoon olive oil
1 teaspoon red wine vinegar
2 teaspoons capers, *chopped*
5 cornichons, *finely chopped*
1 teaspoon Dijon mustard
¼ bunch of parsley, *leaves chopped*
1 organic egg yolk
sea salt and freshly ground black pepper, to taste

1. Coat both sides of the steak with a dusting of sea salt and leave in the fridge for 1 hour.
2. Remove from the fridge and finely chop or mince the steak. Add the olive oil and vinegar and stir through.
3. Fold in the remaining ingredients, or present them separately on a plate. Season to taste with salt and pepper.

Pea Soup with Crickets

This is a fairly classic recipe with some interesting garnishes – purely optional, of course.

SERVES 4

2 tablespoons olive oil
1 onion, *quartered*
4 garlic cloves, *chopped*
4 courgettes, *roughly chopped*
2 bay leaves
4 sprigs of thyme
1 teaspoon dried basil
1.25 litres organic chicken broth or vegetable broth
250g frozen peas
2 tablespoons Spicy Fried Crickets (see recipe page 228)
sea salt and freshly ground black pepper, to taste

1. Place a large saucepan over a medium heat and add the olive oil. Add the onion and garlic and sauté for 3–4 minutes. Add the courgettes, bay leaves, thyme and basil and cook, stirring, for 1–2 minutes, then add the broth.
2. Bring to the boil then reduce the heat to low. Simmer for 5 minutes, then add the peas and cook for a further 5 minutes. Season with salt and pepper and remove from the heat.
3. Allow to cool a little before placing in the blender (a batch at a time, if necessary) and blitzing until smooth. Serve in bowls with a sprinkle of Spicy Fried Crickets, if you like.

The DAS (Delicious Asian Salad)

The dressing on this salad has to be one of my favourites of all time. I highly recommend adjusting it to your preferences and keeping the recipe in your back pocket.

SERVES 2

1 organic chicken breast, *poached, cooled and shredded*
1 red onion, *thinly sliced*
¼ bunch of mint, *leaves picked*
¼ bunch of coriander, *leaves picked*
2 shallots, *chopped*
75g toasted desiccated coconut
1 punnet of cherry tomatoes, *halved*
1 long red chilli, *sliced*
3–4 tablespoons dressing (see below)
2 tablespoons coconut cream
2 organic eggs, *boiled and halved*
sea salt and freshly ground black pepper, to taste

DRESSING

1 garlic clove, *crushed*
1 small red chilli, *finely chopped*
2cm knob of fresh ginger, *finely chopped*
juice of 2 limes
1 teaspoon honey
1 tablespoon fish sauce

1. Combine the ingredients for the dressing in a small jar, cover and shake vigorously. Taste and adjust flavours to your liking.
2. In a large mixing bowl, combine all the ingredients except the dressing, coconut cream and eggs. Lightly toss. Add the dressing and gently toss again.
3. Transfer to a serving plate or bowls, drizzle with the coconut cream, and season with salt and pepper. Serve with the eggs on top.

Chargrilled Courgette Salad

This meat-free salad is to die for (not literally, but it is YUM). It's packed full of rich flavours.

SERVES 2

4 tablespoons olive oil, plus extra for brushing

4 garlic cloves, *chopped*

2 celery stalks, *chopped*

½ bunch of parsley, *stalks finely chopped and leaves roughly chopped*

1 teaspoon chilli flakes

1 tablespoon capers

1 tablespoon red wine vinegar

6 anchovies

3 large courgettes, *cut in half lengthways*

handful pistachios, *crushed*

1 teaspoon grated lemon zest

sea salt and freshly ground black pepper, to taste

1. Place a small frying pan or saucepan over a low heat and add the olive oil. Add the garlic, celery, parsley stalks, chilli flakes, capers, red wine vinegar and anchovies and cook, stirring occasionally, for 10–15 minutes. Remove from the heat and set aside.

2. Heat a griddle pan over a high heat. Brush both sides of the courgettes with a little olive oil.

3. Place the courgettes, flesh side down, on the griddle and cook for 2–3 minutes, or until charred. Remove from the heat, allow to cool, then cut into small wedges.

4. Add the courgettes to the celery mix, sprinkle with the parsley leaves, pistachios and lemon zest, then season with salt and pepper.

Haddock in Caper Butter

Such an easy but delicious meal for lunch or a midweek dinner. From start to finish, it only takes 15 minutes.

SERVES 4

3 tablespoons organic ghee
4 MSC haddock fillets, skin on
2 tablespoons capers
juice of 1–2 lemons
2 handfuls rocket leaves
1 punnet of cherry tomatoes, *halved*
½ bunch of parsley, *leaves roughly chopped*
2 tablespoons olive oil
1 tablespoon red wine vinegar
sea salt and freshly ground black pepper, to taste

1. Place a large frying pan over a high heat and add the ghee. Add the whiting, skin side down, and the capers. Cook for 1 minute before flipping the fish over and cooking for a further 1 minute.
2. Remove from the heat, drizzle the fish with lemon juice and a little caper butter, and season with salt and pepper.
3. In a mixing bowl, combine the rocket, tomatoes, parsley, olive oil and red wine vinegar. Season and serve with the fish.

Leftovers Frittata

A perfect way to use up any leftovers sitting around in the fridge or pantry – there are no rules.

SERVES 4

2 tablespoons organic ghee
1 red onion, *quartered*
2 garlic cloves, *sliced*
6–8 cavolo nero leaves, *stalks removed, chopped*
10 organic eggs, *lightly whisked*
75ml water
400g leftover cooked squash or sweet potato, diced
250g leftover organic lamb or chicken, diced
1 teaspoon dried rosemary
1 teaspoon dried thyme
sea salt and freshly ground black pepper, to taste

1. Preheat your oven to 180°C.
2. Place a frying pan over a medium heat and add the ghee. Add the onion, garlic and kale and sauté for 3–4 minutes, or until softened. Remove from the heat and set aside.
3. In a large mixing bowl, combine the eggs and 75ml of water. Season with salt and pepper.
4. Transfer the onion mixture to a greased baking tray and top with the squash/sweet potato, lamb/chicken and dried herbs. Add the eggs and season with salt and pepper.
5. Bake for 30 minutes, or until browned on top. Remove from the oven and allow to rest for 5 minutes before serving.

Spicy Lamb Larb

SERVES 4

2 tablespoons coconut oil
4cm knob of fresh ginger, *grated or finely chopped*
4 garlic cloves, *finely chopped*
2 shallots, *peeled and chopped*
1 stalk of lemongrass, *white part only, finely chopped*
500g organic lamb mince
1 small red chilli, *chopped*
juice of 2 limes
1 tablespoon gluten-free fish sauce
1 teaspoon honey
¼ bunch of coriander, *leaves chopped*
¼ bunch of mint, *leaves chopped*
sea salt and freshly ground black pepper, to taste

1. Place a large frying pan over a medium heat and add the coconut oil. Add the ginger, garlic and shallots and sauté for 3–4 minutes. Add the lemongrass and continue to cook for 1 minute.
2. Increase the heat to high and add the mince, stirring until browned, then reduce the heat and cook for 8–10 minutes.
3. Meanwhile, combine the chilli, lime juice, fish sauce and honey. Stir, and adjust flavours to your preference.
4. Add the chilli mixture to the lamb and cook for 2 minutes. Remove from the heat and fold in the coriander and mint. Season with salt pepper, and serve.

Cauliflower Bruschetta

The base for this bruschetta can also be used as a low-carb, grain-free pizza base.

SERVES 4

1 whole cauliflower
35g ground almonds
2 organic eggs
3 tablespoons olive oil
1 punnet of medley cherry tomatoes, *halved*
2 tablespoons capers
4 anchovies, *roughly chopped*
½ bunch of basil, *leaves torn*
¼ bunch of parsley, *leaves roughly chopped*
sea salt and freshly ground black pepper, to taste

1. Preheat your oven to 140°C. Line one or two baking trays with baking paper.
2. Roughly chop the cauliflower into florets before popping into a food processor. Blitz until finely chopped.
3. Transfer to the baking tray/s and bake for 15 minutes to dry out. Remove from the oven and allow to cool.
4. Return the cauliflower to the food processor and add the ground almonds, eggs and 1 tablespoon of the olive oil. Season to taste with salt and pepper. Blitz until a dough forms. Remove.
5. Increase the oven temperature to 180°C and form a pizza shape with the dough. Place on a lined baking tray and bake for 25 minutes, or until golden brown.
6. Meanwhile, combine the tomatoes, capers, anchovies, basil, parsley and the remaining olive oil. Season to taste with salt and pepper.
7. Remove the 'bruschetta' from the oven and serve with the tomato salad.

Barbecued Venison

Venison is a sustainable food source in the UK. It is a lean meat, which doesn't tolerate overcooking too well, so aim for rare or medium-rare at most.

SERVES 4

2–3 tablespoons olive oil
2 garlic cloves, *crushed*
1 long red chilli, *chopped*
6 sprigs of lemon thyme, *leaves picked*
1 teaspoon ground cumin
4 wild or grass-fed venison steaks
juice of 1 lemon
sea salt and freshly ground black pepper, to taste

1. Preheat your barbecue to high.
2. In a mixing bowl, combine the olive oil, garlic, chilli, thyme leaves and cumin. Once the barbecue is hot, brush some of the oil on one side of the steaks. Place on the barbecue, brushed side down, and cook for 2–3 minutes (times vary according to the thickness of the steak). Brush the up-facing side with the oil, flip over and cook for a further 2–3 minutes.
3. Remove from the heat and cover lightly with foil. Allow to rest for 2–3 minutes, then slice into 1–2cm slices. Drizzle over the lemon juice, season with salt and pepper, and serve.

Barbecued Lobster with Herb Butter

SERVES 4

2 fresh sustainable lobsters, *halved lengthways*
4–6 tablespoons Herb Butter (see recipe page 249), *melted*
juice of 1 lemon
sea salt and freshly ground black pepper, to taste

1. Heat your barbecue to high.
2. Place the halved lobster, flesh side up, on a baking tray. Brush with some of the Herb Butter.
3. Place the lobster, flesh side down, on the barbecue and cook for 4 minutes, or until charred. Turn over and cook for a further 8–10 minutes while brushing on the butter regularly.
4. Once cooked through, remove the lobster from the barbecue and set aside for 1–2 minutes to rest. Drizzle with lemon juice, season with salt and pepper, and serve.

Crab and Avo Smash

Brown crab from the Inshore Potting Agreement area in Devon, the Western Channel or Cornwall are the best choices for crab in the UK.

SERVES 2

2 avocados
juice of 2 limes
1 tablespoon olive oil
1 teaspoon chilli flakes
½ teaspoon ground cumin
¼ bunch of coriander, *leaves chopped*
200g cooked white crabmeat
1 cucumber, *cut into wedges*
sea salt and freshly ground black pepper, to taste

1. In a large mixing bowl, combine the avocado, lime juice, olive oil, chilli flakes, cumin, fresh coriander and crabmeat. Mash with a fork and season with salt and pepper.
2. Serve with wedges of cucumber.

DINNER

Slow-cooked Lamb with Anchovies

Hands down, slow-cooked lamb is my favourite. I've cooked it a thousand different ways, but this is one of the best.

SERVES 6

2 tablespoons olive oil
1.8–2kg organic lamb shoulder
4 shallots, *peeled and halved*
6 garlic cloves, whole
6 anchovies
2 bay leaves
6 sprigs of thyme
6 sprigs of rosemary
750ml organic beef or chicken broth
sea salt and freshly ground black pepper, to taste

1. Preheat your oven to 200°C.
2. Place an ovenproof dish over a high heat and add the olive oil. Add the lamb shoulder and cook, turning regularly, until browned. Remove from the heat.
3. Return the ovenproof dish to a low heat and add the shallots, garlic, anchovies, bay leaves, thyme, rosemary and broth.
4. Season with salt and pepper, pop the lid on and place in the oven. Reduce the heat to 130°C and cook for 5–6 hours. At the 4-hour mark, check to see if more broth or water is required.
5. Once the lamb is falling off the bone, remove from the oven and allow to rest for 10 minutes. Adjust seasonings and serve.

Beef Cheeks

One of my favourite cuts of meat, and one that features on my restaurant menus – it's moist and full of flavour.

SERVES 6-8

2 tablespoons organic tallow or ghee

4 x 450g grass-fed/-finished beef cheeks

6 shallots, *peeled and halved*

4 garlic cloves

6 bay leaves

1 tablespoon caraway seeds

1 tablespoon cumin seeds

4 cloves

2 star anise

125ml red wine

750ml organic beef bone broth

sea salt and freshly ground black pepper, to taste

1. Preheat your oven to 220°C.
2. Place a large casserole dish over a high heat and add the tallow or ghee. Add the beef cheeks and brown all over, turning often. Remove from the dish and set aside, retaining the fat in the pan.
3. Reduce the heat to medium and add the shallots and garlic. Cook for 3–4 minutes, then add the bay leaves, caraway seeds, cumin seeds, cloves and star anise, stirring for 2–3 minutes.
4. Increase the temperature to high and add the red wine. Cook long enough for the alcohol to evaporate (1–2 minutes). Reduce the heat to medium and return the beef to the dish, along with the broth. Season with salt and pepper and bring to a simmer.
5. Pop the lid on and place in the oven. Reduce the heat to 160°C and cook the cheeks for 4–5 hours, turning once, or until the cheeks fall apart.
6. Remove from the oven and allow to rest for 20 minutes. Adjust seasonings and serve.

Cod Curry

There's something incredibly comforting about a rich yellow fish curry. It's like having a cuddle from someone you love.

SERVES 4

4 garlic cloves, *chopped*

4 small green chillies, *chopped*

2 teaspoons chopped fresh ginger

2 teaspoons chopped fresh turmeric

2 tablespoons coconut oil

1 red onion, *sliced*

2 teaspoons ground coriander

1 teaspoon ground cumin

2 teaspoons ground turmeric

15 fresh curry leaves

250ml fish stock

1 x 400ml can coconut milk

1 tablespoon gluten-free fish sauce

200g green beans, *trimmed*

750g MSC cod, *chopped into large chunks*

½ bunch of coriander, *leaves roughly chopped*

juice of 1 lime

sea salt and freshly ground black pepper, to taste

1. Place the garlic, chilli, ginger and fresh turmeric in a mortar and pestle and pound to a paste.

2. Place a deep-sided frying pan over a medium heat and add the coconut oil. Add the onion and fry for 2–3 minutes. Add the garlic paste and fry for 3–4 minutes. Add the ground coriander, cumin and turmeric and continue to fry for 2–3 minutes (add a little more coconut oil if needed).

3. Add the curry leaves, fish stock and coconut milk, bring to a simmer and cook for 10 minutes. Add the fish sauce and stir in. Add the green beans and cook for 2–3 minutes.

4. Place the cod in the pan and cook for 4–5 minutes, or until the fish is cooked through. Remove from the heat, stir through the coriander leaves and lime juice, and season with salt and pepper. Serve.

Lamb and Roasted Squash Curry

Perfect for an autumn or winter's evening . . . and pretty good in spring and summer, too!

SERVES 4

1 kg butternut squash, *unpeeled, cut into 2–3cm chunks*
4 tablespoons ground cumin
4 tablespoons coconut oil
200g organic butter or ghee
3 onions, *quartered*
4 garlic cloves, *chopped*
4 long red chillies, *chopped*
2 x 400g tins chopped tomatoes
2 tablespoons ground turmeric
2 tablespoons ground coriander
3 tablespoons sweet paprika
300ml vegetable stock or water
500g organic lamb leg, *diced*
400ml coconut cream
½ bunch of coriander, leaves chopped
sea salt and freshly ground black pepper, to taste

1. Heat your oven to 180°C.

2. Arrange the squash, skin side down, on a baking tray, dust with 1 tablespoon of the cumin and drizzle over the coconut oil. Roast for 45 minutes, or until golden.

3. Place a large saucepan over a medium heat and add the butter. Add the onions, garlic and chillies and cook, stirring, for 3–4 minutes. Add the tomatoes, remaining spices, stock or water and diced lamb, and season with salt and pepper. Bring to the boil, then reduce the heat and simmer for 1¼ hours, or until the lamb is tender.

4. Transfer the roast squash to the saucepan and cook until the squash has warmed through. Remove from the heat and stir in the coconut cream and chopped coriander. Adjust seasonings and serve.

One-pot Chicken

This is exactly my style of cooking – fuss-free yet delicious!

SERVES 4

2 tablespoons organic ghee
6 anchovies, *roughly chopped*
1 teaspoon chilli flakes
2 tablespoons capers
3 garlic cloves, *chopped*
6 sprigs of thyme
2 teaspoons dried oregano
grated zest of 1 lemon
500g organic chicken thigh fillets
1 punnet of cherry vine tomatoes
2 tablespoons olive oil
sea salt and freshly ground black pepper, to taste

1. Preheat your oven to 190°C.
2. In a mixing bowl, combine the ghee, anchovies, chilli flakes, capers, garlic, thyme, oregano and lemon zest, and salt and pepper to taste. Add the chicken and mix to coat.
3. Transfer the chicken and seasonings to a baking tray and bake for 20 minutes. Remove from the oven and add the cherry tomatoes, drizzle with the olive oil, then bake for a further 25 minutes.
4. Once the chicken is cooked through, remove from the oven and allow to rest on a board for 5 minutes. Season again with salt and pepper and serve.

Liver and Potatoes

This works well as an appetiser, or you can upsize the quantities and add some extra greens to make it a more substantial dish.

SERVES 4

400g organic calf's liver, *trimmed and chopped*
2 tablespoons organic ghee
250g new potatoes, *quatered*
¼ bunch of parsley, *stalks finely chopped, leaves roughly chopped*
2 large chard leaves, *stalks removed, roughly chopped*
1 red onion, *sliced*
juice of 1 lemon
1 teaspoon sumac
sea salt and freshly ground black pepper, to taste

1. Soak the liver in water or milk for 1 hour, rinse and pat dry.
2. Place a frying pan over a high heat and add 1 tablespoon of the ghee. Add the potatoes and cook, tossing often, for 2–3 minutes, or until colouration occurs.
3. Add the parsley stalks and liver and cook for 2 minutes. Add the remaining ghee, then add the chard. Toss well and cook for 1–2 minutes. Remove from the heat, season with salt and pepper, and allow to rest.
4. Meanwhile, in a mixing bowl, combine the onion, lemon juice, parsley leaves and sumac and toss together. Serve over the livers and season again with salt and pepper, if desired.

Sausage Hotpot

Good-quality sausages are a non-negotiable, and fortunately the range of organic and grass-fed/-finished sausages is on the rise.

SERVES 4

8 gluten-free organic sausages
2 tablespoons olive oil
1 onion, *sliced*
4 garlic cloves, *crushed*
6 sprigs of rosemary
6 sprigs of thyme
2 teaspoons caraway seeds
2 carrots, *sliced*
500ml organic beef bone broth
2 tablespoons tomato purée
600g tinned chopped tomatoes
¼ head of cauliflower, *cut into florets*
¼ bunch of parsley, *leaves roughly chopped*
sea salt and freshly ground black pepper, to taste

1. Place a large frying pan over a high heat, add the sausages and fry until browned (they don't have to be cooked through at this stage). Remove from the heat and set aside.

2. Preheat your oven to 180°C.

3. Place a large ovenproof dish over a medium heat and add the olive oil. Add the onion and garlic and sauté for 3–4 minutes. Add the rosemary, thyme and caraway seeds and stir for 1 minute. Add the carrots and stir for 1 minute.

4. Add the beef broth and increase the heat to high. Cook until 75 per cent of the broth has evaporated, then add the tomato purée and diced tomatoes.

5. Cut the sausages into 2cm pieces and transfer to the casserole. Add the cauliflower, pop the lid on and bake in the oven for 25 minutes.

6. Remove from the oven and season with salt and pepper. Fold in the parsley just before serving.

Salmon Curry

Cooking curries that require making paste from scratch can seem intimidating, but it's no stress, really, as long as you have a good stock of herbs in the pantry. Make double, triple or quadruple the quantity and freeze in portions for future use.

SERVES 4

3 garlic cloves, *roughly chopped*
4cm knob of ginger, *roughly chopped*
2 small red chillies, *roughly chopped*
1 tablespoon madras curry powder
2 teaspoons whole coriander seeds
2 teaspoons panch phoran (Indian five-spice blend)
2 tablespoons coconut oil
1 onion, *quartered*
4–5 large tomatoes, *roughly chopped*
10 fresh curry leaves
300ml coconut milk
600g skinless MSC salmon, *cut into 3cm pieces*
sea salt
¼ bunch of coriander, *leaves roughly chopped*
2 tablespoons shredded coconut
juice of 1 lime

1. In a mortar and pestle, combine the garlic, ginger, chillies and spices and grind until a paste is formed.
2. Place a large frying pan over a medium heat and add the coconut oil. Add the onion and fry for 2–3 minutes. Add the curry paste and stir for 2–3 minutes. Add the tomatoes and curry leaves and cook for 3–4 minutes.
3. Add the coconut milk and bring to a simmer, stirring often. Add the chopped salmon and cook for 5 minutes, or until the fish is cooked through. Add salt to taste.
4. Remove from the heat, add the coriander leaves and fold through. Serve topped with shredded coconut and lime juice.

Chicken Cacciatore

SERVES 4

2 tablespoons olive oil
500g organic chicken thigh fillets, skin on
1 onion, *quartered*
4 garlic cloves, *chopped*
2 teaspoons dried rosemary
250ml red wine
1 x 400g tin chopped tomatoes
1 red pepper, *roughly chopped*
20 pitted green olives
¼ bunch of parsley, *leaves roughly chopped*
sea salt and freshly ground black pepper, to taste

1. Place a large frying pan over a medium–high heat and add 1 tablespoon of the olive oil. Add the chicken, skin-side down, and fry for 3–4 minutes, or until browned. Turn the chicken over and fry for 2–3 minutes. Remove from the heat and set aside.
2. Reduce the heat to medium and add the remaining olive oil to the pan. Add the onion and garlic and sauté for 2–3 minutes. Add the rosemary and cook, stirring, for 1 minute.
3. Turn the heat to high, add the red wine and allow the alcohol to evaporate (1–2 minutes). Add the tomatoes, pepper and olives and pop the chicken back into the pan. Reduce the heat to medium and continue to cook for 15 minutes, or until the chicken is cooked through.
4. Remove from the heat and fold through the parsley. Season with salt and pepper, and serve.

Burger Patties

It's totally fine to use one type of mince for your burgers; however, combining three different cuts ensures greater fat and flavour content.

SERVES 4

600g grass-fed/-finished mince (⅓ chuck, ⅓ brisket, ⅓ short rib)
2 garlic cloves, *crushed*
½ brown onion, *finely chopped*
1 tablespoon Dijon mustard
1 teaspoon dried oregano
½ teaspoon chilli flakes
1 tablespoon organic ghee
2 tomatoes, *sliced, to serve*
2 tablespoons mayonnaise, *to serve*
4 gherkins, *sliced, to serve*
jalapeños, *to serve*
sea salt and freshly ground black pepper, to taste

1. Combine the mince, garlic, onion, mustard, oregano and chilli flakes in a large bowl. Season with salt and pepper.
2. Divide and shape the mixture into 4 patties. Set aside.
3. Place a frying pan over a high heat and add the ghee. Add the patties and cook for 3–4 minutes on each side, or until cooked through and crisp on the outside. Remove from heat and allow to rest for 2 minutes.
4. Serve the patties with sliced tomatoes, mayo, gherkins and jalapeños.

Pesto Meatballs

Mince is versatile and affordable, useful when cooking for the family.

SERVES 4

500g grass-fed/-finished beef mince
1 organic egg
2 onions, *chopped*
4 garlic cloves, *chopped*
3–4 tablespoons Pesto (see recipe page 241)
2 tablespoons olive oil
1 teaspoon dried oregano
1 x 400g tin chopped tomatoes
400g tomato passata
1 tablespoon organic butter
small handful of basil leaves
sea salt and freshly ground black pepper, to taste

1. In a large mixing bowl, combine the mince, egg, half the onions, half the garlic and all the pesto. Season to taste with salt and pepper.

2. Use your hands to mix the ingredients thoroughly, then shape into meatballs – the size is totally up to you (cooking times will vary). Set aside.

3. Place a large saucepan over a medium heat and add the olive oil. Add the remaining onions and garlic, plus the oregano, and cook for 3–4 minutes, or until the onion has softened. Add the diced tomatoes and passata and bring to a simmer.

4. Meanwhile, place a large frying pan over a high heat and add the butter. Place the meatballs in the pan and cook until browned all over. Transfer to the simmering tomato sauce.

5. Cook the meatballs for a further 6 minutes, or until cooked through. Tear up the basil leaves and gently stir in. Adjust seasonings. Serve.

Venison Bolognese

SERVES 4

3 tablespoons olive oil

2 shallots, *peeled and quartered*

4 garlic cloves, *chopped*

1 celery stalk, *chopped*

2 bay leaves

2 teaspoons dried oregano

1 teaspoon dried basil

1 teaspoon dried rosemary

500g wild or grass-fed venison mince

500ml organic beef bone broth

1 large carrot, *grated*

600g tinned chopped tomatoes

100g tomato purée

2 large courgettes, *spiralised*

sea salt and freshly ground black pepper, to taste

1. Place a large saucepan over a medium heat and add 2 tablespoons of the olive oil. Add the shallots, garlic and celery and sauté for 3–4 minutes. Add the bay leaves and dried herbs and stir for 1–2 minutes.
2. Add the mince and turn the heat up to high. Brown the mince, stirring. Add the broth and cook until 75 per cent of the liquid has evaporated.
3. Add the carrot, diced tomatoes and tomato purée and stir well. Bring to the boil, then reduce to a simmer and cook for 25 minutes, or until reduced to your liking.
4. Remove the bolognese from the heat. Dress the courgette noodles with the remaining olive oil and season with salt and pepper. Serve the noodles folded into the sauce.

Fish Provençale

I was incredibly lucky to grow up in pubs. Mum and Dad were always creating new dishes for the customers. One of the best 'specials of the day' was chicken or fish Provençale. Gurnard has become more popular recently as a sustainable fish option.

SERVES 2

1–2 tablespoons olive oil
1 brown onion, *sliced*
2 garlic cloves, *chopped*
¼ bunch of parsley, *stalks finely chopped, leaves roughly chopped*
1 teaspoon herbes de Provence
100ml white wine
1 tablespoon tomato purée
300g tinned chopped tomatoes
1 roasted pepper, *skin removed, sliced*
8–10 pitted kalamata olives
2 whole gurnards, descaled and gutted
1 tablespoon organic butter
juice of ½ lemon
sea salt and freshly ground black pepper, to taste

1. Preheat your oven to 190°C.
2. Place a saucepan over a medium heat and add the olive oil. Add the onion, garlic and parsley stalks and sauté for 3–4 minutes. Add the herbes de Provence and stir for 1 minute.
3. Add the white and allow the alcohol to evaporate (1–2 minutes). Add the tomato purée, tinned tomatoes, pepper and olives and bring to a gentle simmer.
4. Place the fish on a baking tray and add the butter. Season with salt and pepper and bake, lightly covered with foil, for 30–40 minutes, depending on the size of the fish.
5. Transfer to a serving dish and drizzle with the lemon juice. Season the tomato sauce with salt and pepper and pour over the fish. Sprinkle with parsley leaves, and serve.

Sage and Chicken Livers

SERVES 4

2 tablespoons organic butter
6 sage leaves
1 tablespoon capers
400g organic chicken livers, *trimmed and chopped*
juice of 1 lemon
sea salt and freshly ground black pepper, to taste

1. Place a large frying pan over a high heat, add the butter, sage and capers and fry for 1 minute. Add the chicken livers and fry for 3–4 minutes, or until browned and cooked through. Remove from the heat and allow to rest.
2. Drizzle with the lemon juice, season with salt and pepper, and serve.

Confit Salmon

In my restaurants, I confit most of our proteins. It's a great way to cook meat or fish, as it helps to retain moisture. The end result is always succulent.

SERVES 4

500ml olive oil or 500g organic ghee
½ bulb of garlic
grated zest of 1 lemon
10 sprigs of lemon thyme
½ bunch of dill
4 x 120g MSC salmon fillets, *skin removed*
sea salt and freshly ground black pepper, to taste

1. Place a frying pan (or roasting tin small enough to snugly fit the salmon) over a low heat and add the olive oil or ghee. Add the garlic, lemon zest, thyme and dill and gently heat for 10 minutes to allow the flavours to infuse.
2. Increase the temperature slightly until very small bubbles appear in the oil. Place the fillets in the oil and cook for 8–10 minutes. Remove the pan from the heat and allow the fillets to rest in the oil for 5 minutes.
3. Remove from the oil, season with salt and pepper, and serve.

Midweek Mince and Aubergine

SERVES 4

1 tablespoon olive oil

1 onion, *chopped*

4 garlic cloves, *chopped*

1 carrot, *chopped*

1 celery stalk, *chopped*

2 teaspoons dried oregano

1 teaspoon dried basil

250ml red wine

500g grass-fed/-finished beef mince

1 x 400g tinned chopped tomatoes

400g tomato passata

1 aubergine, *cut into 1cm cubes*

sea salt and freshly ground black pepper, to taste

1. Place a large frying pan over a medium heat and add the olive oil. Add the onion, garlic, carrot and celery and sauté for 4–5 minutes, or until the vegetables have softened. Add the oregano and basil and cook for 1–2 minutes, stirring.
2. Increase the heat to high and add the red wine. Allow the alcohol to evaporate (1–2 minutes) before adding the mince. Brown the mince, stirring often.
3. Add the tinned tomatoes and passata and simmer for 20 minutes. Add the aubergine and cook for a further 5 minutes.
4. Season with salt and pepper, and serve.

Roast Butterfly Chicken with Harissa

Serve with some yummy greens or roasted veggies, such as
blanched dandelion greens.

SERVES 4

1 teaspoon coriander seeds
4 garlic cloves
1 tablespoon harissa paste
½ preserved lemon, *finely chopped*
2 tablespoons organic ghee
1 teaspoon sumac
1 organic chicken, *butterflied*
juice of ½ lemon
sea salt and freshly ground black pepper, to taste

1. Using a mortar and pestle, smash the coriander seeds. Add the garlic
   cloves and continue to pound. Add the harissa paste, preserved
   lemon, ghee and sumac. Combine ingredients well.
2. Place the chicken in a large dish and massage the marinade into
   the skin. Place a lid over the dish and refrigerate for a minimum of
   2 hours.
3. Remove the chicken from the fridge 20 minutes prior to cooking.
   Preheat your oven to 200°C or barbecue to high.
4. Place the chicken in a roasting tin and put into the oven, or place
   onto the hot grill of the barbecue, and cook for 25 minutes.
   Turn and cook for a further 15 minutes, or until cooked through.
   Remove from the heat and allow to rest, covered loosely with foil,
   for 5 minutes.
5. Drizzle with lemon juice, season with salt and pepper, and serve.

Rachel's Chicken Soup with Preserved Lemon

Gotta say, my mum-in-law is a whizz in the kitchen. She's actually a whizz at everything. This is her chook and preserved lemon recipe.

SERVES 4

2 tablespoons olive oil
1 large onion, *diced*
6 garlic cloves, *chopped*
2 carrots, *diced*
2 celery stalks, *diced*
½ preserved lemon, *roughly chopped*
1 organic chicken
1 litre organic vegetable or chicken broth
300g potatoes, *washed and chopped into large chunks* (optional)
2 large handfuls of chopped spinach or chard
sea salt and freshly ground black pepper, to taste

1. Place a large saucepan over a medium heat and add the olive oil. Add the onion, garlic, carrot and celery and sauté for 5–6 minutes. Add the preserved lemon and stir.

2. Place the whole chicken in the saucepan and pour in the broth. Bring to the boil, then reduce the heat to low and simmer, with the lid on, for 1½ hours, or until the chicken falls off the bone. If using potatoes, add once the broth has simmered for 50 minutes.

3. Remove from the heat and add the spinach or chard. Stir for 1–2 minutes.

4. Take the chicken out of the soup and strip the meat from the carcass. Return the meat to the soup, season with salt and pepper, and serve.

Slow-cooked Roast Pigeon

Mum and Dad used to put pigeon pie on the specials board in their pubs. The customers loved it. You can ask your friendly local butcher for pigeon.

SERVES 4

2 tablespoons olive oil
4 shallots, *peeled and halved*
2 carrots, *sliced*
4 garlic cloves
6 sprigs of rosemary
2 sage leaves
2 bay leaves
4 organic pigeons (squab)
125ml white wine
750ml organic chicken broth
sea salt and freshly ground black pepper, to taste

1. Preheat your oven to 200°C.
2. Place an ovenproof dish over a medium heat and add the olive oil. Add the shallots, carrots and garlic and sauté for 3–4 minutes. Add the rosemary, sage and bay leaves and stir for 1 minute.
3. Turn the heat to high and add the pigeons. Brown the birds, turning often, for 3–5 minutes, then add the wine and allow to reduce by half. Add the chicken broth and season with salt and pepper.
4. Place the lid on the dish and pop in the oven. Reduce the temperature to 140°C and cook for 3–4 hours, or until the meat falls away from the bone. Remove from the oven, adjust seasonings, and serve.

Steak with Buttery Mushrooms

This is a rich, earthy and ballsy dish. If you're after something light and refreshing, keep browsing.

SERVES 4

2 grass-fed/-finished rump steaks
100g organic butter, plus 1 tablespoon, extra
1 teaspoon fresh or dried tarragon
1 teaspoon fresh or dried thyme
2 garlic cloves, *crushed*
1 large portobello mushroom, *sliced*
2 oyster mushrooms, *quartered*
8 chestnut mushrooms, *halved*
2 teaspoons lemon juice
sea salt and freshly ground black pepper, to taste

1. Remove the steaks from the fridge 30 minutes prior to cooking.
2. Place a large frying pan over a medium heat and add the 100g of butter. Add the tarragon, thyme and garlic and cook for 3–4 minutes. Add the mushrooms and cook for 6–7 minutes, or until softened and browned.
3. Remove from the heat, add 1 teaspoon of the lemon juice and season with salt and pepper. Transfer to a bowl.
4. Heat a frying pan over a high heat, add the remaining butter, season the steak and place in the pan. Cook the steaks for 3 minutes on each side, or until done to your liking. Remove from the heat and allow to rest for 4–5 minutes.
5. Cut the steaks into strips and drizzle over the remaining lemon juice. Add the mushrooms, season and serve.

Easy Moroccan Chicken

SERVES 4

200g unsweetened coconut yoghurt
2 tablespoons lime juice
2 tablespoons Moroccan spice or ras el hanout
1 organic chicken, *butterflied*
2–3 tablespoons olive oil
sea salt and freshly ground black pepper, to taste

1. In a large mixing bowl, combine the coconut yoghurt, lime juice and Moroccan spice. Season to taste with salt and pepper.
2. Add the chicken and coat entirely, then leave to marinate in the fridge for at least 2 hours.
3. Preheat your oven to 180°C and heat a griddle pan over a high heat.
4. Place the chicken in the pan, skin side down, and cook for 5 minutes. Turn and cook for a further 5 minutes. Transfer to a baking tray, drizzle with olive oil and put in the oven for 35–40 minutes, or until cooked through.
5. Remove from the oven, season and serve.

Lamb Mince with Squash and Mushrooms

This is a prime example of how comfort food can be healthy. Phew!

SERVES 4

2 tablespoons olive oil
2 onions, *chopped*
4 garlic cloves, *chopped*
1 teaspoon ground cumin
1 teaspoon cinnamon
2 tablespoons fresh or dried rosemary
500g organic lamb mince
½ butternut squash, *peeled and chopped into 1cm cubes*
500ml organic beef bone broth
250g chestnut mushrooms, *quartered*
sea salt and freshly ground black pepper, to taste

1. Place a frying pan over a medium heat and add the olive oil. Add the onions and garlic and sauté for 3–4 minutes. Add the cumin, cinnamon and rosemary and cook, stirring, for 2–3 minutes.
2. Increase the heat and add the mince. Once browned, add the squash and beef broth, reduce the heat to low and simmer for 20 minutes.
3. Add the mushrooms and continue to cook for 10 minutes, or until the squash is tender. Season with salt and pepper, and serve.

Barbecued Rabbit

The UK has a plethora of game meat to cook with, such as venison and rabbit. Choosing local meats such as these helps to reduce the ecological cost of transporting imported meat.

SERVES 4

2 tablespoons olive oil
2 garlic cloves, *crushed*
1 teaspoon capers
3 anchovies, *roughly chopped*
1 tablespoon dried rosemary
4 rabbit legs
juice of ½ lemon
sea salt and freshly ground black pepper, to taste

1. In a mixing bowl, combine the oil, garlic, capers, anchovies and rosemary. Add the rabbit pieces, mix well and leave to marinate while you heat your barbecue.
2. Heat your barbecue to high. Season the rabbit legs with salt and pepper.
3. Place the rabbit legs on the barbecue and cook for 35–40 minutes, turning every so often. Baste the meat continuously with the marinade.
4. Once cooked to your liking, remove from the heat, cover loosely with foil and allow to rest for 3–5 minutes.
5. Drizzle with lemon juice, season again with salt and pepper, and serve.

Roast Venison

Wild venison is available at your local butcher's or can be ordered online. It's also a sustainable meat source in the UK. Serve this with roasted potatoes and herb mayonnaise.

SERVES 4

3 tablespoons organic butter or ghee
1 teaspoon chilli flakes
1kg venison roasting joint
6 sprigs of rosemary
sea salt and freshly ground black pepper, to taste

1. Preheat your oven to 200°C.
2. Combine the butter/ghee and chilli flakes.
3. Place a frying pan over a high heat and add the butter mixture. Place the venison in the pan and brown the meat by rotating it every 20–30 seconds until the entire shoulder is browned. Reserve the butter.
4. Place the sprigs of rosemary on the bottom of a small roasting tin. Transfer the venison to the tin and pour the butter over. Roast for 25 minutes.
5. Remove from the oven and allow to rest, lightly covered with foil, for 5 minutes. Slice, season with salt and pepper, and serve.

Marinated Pork

Free-range pork is now available in some UK supermarkets, or ask your friendly local butcher.

SERVES 4

2 garlic cloves, *minced*
juice of 2–3 limes
1 tablespoon honey
3 tablespoons olive oil
1 teaspoon chilli powder
2 pork fillets, *cut into medallions*
sea salt and freshly ground black pepper, to taste

1. In a mixing bowl, combine the garlic, lime juice, honey, olive oil and chilli powder, and salt and pepper to taste. Add the pork medallions and allow to marinate for 2 hours in the fridge.
2. Bring the meat to room temperature, then place a frying pan or griddle pan over a high heat. Add the pork, removing any excess marinade, and cook for 3 minutes on each side, or until done to your liking.
3. Remove from the heat, allow to rest for 5 minutes, then season with salt and pepper and serve.

Fuss-free Fish Stew

Try saying that three times quickly! You can use fresh or frozen seafood for this recipe.

SERVES 4

3 tablespoons olive oil

1 red onion, *sliced*

3 garlic cloves, *chopped*

½ bunch of parsley, *stalks finely chopped, leaves roughly chopped*

1 teaspoon smoked paprika

½ teaspoon sweet paprika

½ teaspoon chilli flakes

1 x 400g tin chopped tomatoes

750ml organic vegetable or chicken broth

1 tablespoon red wine vinegar

400g MSC white fish (such as cod or haddock), *chopped*

150g MSC raw prawns, *peeled*

2 large handfuls of baby spinach leaves

sea salt and freshly ground black pepper, to taste

1. Place a large saucepan over a medium heat and add the olive oil. Add the onion, garlic and parsley stalks and sauté for 3–4 minutes. Add the spices and fry for a further 1 minute.

2. Add the chopped tomatoes, vegetable or chicken broth and the red wine vinegar. Bring to the boil, then reduce to a simmer and cook for 8 minutes.

3. Add the fish and cook for 4–5 minutes. Add the prawns and cook until opaque (about 3–4 minutes).

4. Add the spinach and parsley leaves and stir through. Remove from the heat, season with salt and pepper, and serve.

Porchetta

Pork belly would be in my top five cuts of meat of all time. Pork belly for breakfast, I say!

SERVES 8

2kg rolled boneless organic/free-range pork belly
4 garlic cloves, *crushed*
2 teaspoons grated lemon zest
1 tablespoon fennel seeds
2 teaspoons caraway seeds
1 tablespoon dried rosemary
1 tablespoon coconut oil
sea salt

1. Untie the pork and place on a rack in the sink. Pour boiling water over the skin, then pat dry with a clean tea towel. Place in the fridge, uncovered, for 24 hours to help dry the skin out.

2. Combine the garlic, lemon zest, fennel seeds, caraway seeds, rosemary and coconut oil in a mortar and pestle or a food processor. Grind or whizz to a rough paste. Set aside.

3. Score the pork skin at 1cm intervals. Spread the garlic paste evenly over the flesh side of the meat. Roll and tie up the pork at 2cm increments. Season liberally with sea salt, transfer to a baking tray and leave in the fridge for a minimum of 4 hours.

4. Preheat your oven to 250°C. Roast the pork for 30–35 minutes, or until the skin has crackled. Reduce the heat to 120°C and roast for a further 2 hours, or until cooked through.

5. Remove from the oven and allow to rest for 5 minutes before slicing and serving.

SIDES

Cucumber and Yoghurt

Simple and delicious!

SERVES 2-4

200g unsweetened coconut yoghurt
1 garlic clove, *crushed*
½ bunch of mint, *leaves chopped*
1 tablespoon lemon juice
grated zest of ½ lemon
4 cucumbers, *sliced lengthways*
1 tablespoon macadamia oil
sea salt and freshly ground black pepper, to taste

1. In a large mixing bowl, combine the yoghurt, garlic, mint, lemon juice and lemon zest. Drizzle with the macadamia oil, then season with salt and pepper.
2. Serve with the cucumbers.

Sautéed Veggies

I stayed at a hotel on a recent trip to the United Arab Emirates, and after a few days of the breakfast buffet I was drawn to this dish - simple but tasty.

SERVES 4

3 tablespoons organic ghee
2 garlic cloves, *crushed*
4 carrots, *chopped*
1 teaspoon dried or fresh rosemary
1 teaspoon dried or fresh thyme
2 red onions, *chopped*
2 fennel bulbs, *trimmed and sliced*
4 small courgettes, *chopped*
sea salt and freshly ground black pepper, to taste

1. Place a large frying pan over a medium heat and add the ghee. Add the garlic and cook for 1 minute, stirring.
2. Add the carrots and stir well to coat with ghee. Add the herbs and stir.
3. Add the onions and cook for 2–3 minutes. Add the fennel and cook for a further 2–3 minutes. Add the courgettes and cook until soft.
4. Season with salt and pepper, and serve.

Crispy Rosemary Potatoes with Mayo

I started making these at home for the family and now I'm serving them in my restaurant. They're crisp and delicious.

SERVES 4

160ml organic ghee, *melted*
1 tablespoon dried rosemary
1 teaspoon dried thyme
800g new potatoes, *washed*
sea salt
4–6 tablespoons Horseradish Mayo (see recipe page 244)

1. Preheat your oven to 200°C.
2. Pour the ghee into a baking tray and stir in the rosemary and thyme. Place in the oven for 10 minutes.
3. Meanwhile, bring a saucepan of salted water to the boil, add the potatoes and boil for 10 minutes. Drain, place the lid on the pan and shake vigorously for 10 seconds to rough up the surface of the potatoes.
4. Remove the baking tray from the oven and pop the potatoes in. Use a spatula to coat them with the ghee and herb mixture. Roast for 40 minutes, or until the potatoes are crisp and golden brown.
5. Remove from the oven, sprinkle with sea salt and serve with Horseradish Mayo.

Spicy Fried Crickets

The first time I had crickets was back in 2013 and I found them surprisingly easy to eat. You can order crickets online or from specialty stores.

SERVES 1

150g coconut oil
1 teaspoon ground cumin
1 teaspoon smoked paprika
1 teaspoon sweet paprika
½ teaspoon cayenne pepper
½ teaspoon sumac
250g crickets
sea salt

1. Place a large frying pan or wok over a high heat and add the coconut oil. Add the spices and stir, then add the crickets and cook for 4–5 minutes, or until golden and crisp.
2. Sieve the crickets from the oil and place on paper towels to further drain. Dust with sea salt and serve.

Roasted Buttered Mushrooms

Twice a year my son goes foraging for mushrooms in the Blue Mountains, near Sydney, and brings home a bagful of delicious pine mushrooms. Don't worry if you can't obtain pine mushrooms; portobello mushrooms will work just as well.

SERVES 4

4 pine or portobello mushrooms, *stalks trimmed*
50g organic butter
4 garlic cloves, *crushed*
¼ bunch of parsley, *leaves chopped*
8 sprigs of thyme
juice of 1 lemon
sea salt and freshly ground black pepper, to taste

1. Preheat your oven to 180°C.
2. Place the mushrooms, undersides up, on a baking tray lined with baking paper.
3. In a mixing bowl, combine the butter, garlic and parsley. Rub equal amounts of this butter on each mushroom and place 2 sprigs of thyme on each mushroom. Season with salt and pepper, cover lightly with foil and roast for 15–20 minutes.
4. Remove from the oven, drizzle with lemon juice, season with salt and pepper, and serve.

Delicious Baked Squash with Herbed Oil

SERVES 4

3 tablespoons olive oil
2 teaspoons ground cumin
2 butternut squash, *unpeeled, cut into large chunks*
sea salt and freshly ground black pepper, to taste

HERBED OIL

100ml olive oil
1 long red chilli, *deseeded and finely chopped*
4 sprigs of thyme, *leaves picked*
4 sprigs of rosemary, *leaves picked*
2 garlic cloves, *crushed*

1. Preheat your oven to 200°C. Line one or two baking trays with baking paper.
2. In a bowl, combine the 3 tablespoons of olive oil with the cumin. Season with salt and pepper.
3. Place the chopped squash on the baking tray/s and pour over the oil mixture. Use your hands to ensure the squash is thoroughly coated. Season again and bake for 50 minutes, or until golden and cooked through.
4. Meanwhile, make the herbed oil by combining all the ingredients in a small jar. Cover and shake vigorously. Set aside.
5. Remove the squash from the oven and transfer to a serving bowl or plate. Drizzle with the herbed oil, season with salt and pepper, and serve.

Pan-fried Greens

SERVES 2

1 tablespoon organic ghee
1 tablespoon olive oil
1 teaspoon chilli flakes
1 bunch of tenderstem broccoli, *trimmed*
6 cavelo nero leaves, *roughly chopped*
80g frozen peas
juice of ½ lemon
sea salt and freshly ground black pepper, to taste
1 organic egg, *fried* (optional)

1. Place a large frying pan over a high heat and add the ghee and olive oil. Add the chilli flakes and broccoli and fry for 3–4 minutes, or until lightly charred. Add the cavelo nero and peas and cook for a further 2–3 minutes, or until the peas are warmed through. Remove from the heat.
2. Transfer the greens to a serving dish, drizzle with lemon juice, season with salt and pepper, and serve.
3. If including the egg, add 1 tablespoon of olive oil/ghee to a small frying pan over a medium heat. Crack an egg into the pan and cook through. Add to your serving dish.

Roasted Brussels Sprouts

This is a great side dish or additional element to a roast vegetable salad.

SERVES 4

4–5 teaspoons coconut oil
4 garlic cloves, *crushed*
1 teaspoon chilli flakes
600g Brussels sprouts, *trimmed and halved*
juice of 1 lemon
sea salt and freshly ground black pepper, to taste

1. Preheat your oven to 220°C.
2. Place a large frying pan or ovenproof dish over a medium–high heat and add the coconut oil. Add the garlic and chilli flakes and place the Brussels sprouts cut-side down in the pan. Fry for 5–6 minutes, or until the sprouts begin to brown.
3. Transfer to the oven and bake until crisp and cooked through, about 20 minutes. Toss once or twice during the cooking time.
4. To serve, drizzle with lemon juice and season with salt and pepper.

Sautéed Wild Mushrooms

The combination of mushrooms, butter, salt and lemon is hard to beat. This is a great side dish. Add some chopped chorizo or sausage for something more substantial.

SERVES 4

1kg mixed mushrooms, e.g. shiitake, portobello, porcini, oyster
4 tablespoons organic butter or ghee
2 shallots, *peeled and halved*
4 garlic cloves, *crushed*
50ml white wine
juice of 1 lemon
sea salt and freshly ground black pepper, to taste

1. Slice the mushrooms to approximately the same thickness.
2. Place a large frying pan over a medium–high heat and add the butter or ghee. Add the shallots and sauté for 3–4 minutes. Add the mushrooms and garlic and fry for 5–6 minutes, or until slightly softened.
3. Turn the heat up and add the white wine. Allow the alcohol to evaporate (1–2 minutes). Reduce the heat and continue to fry until the liquid has reduced and the mushrooms have browned.
4. Remove from the heat, drizzle with lemon juice, season with salt and pepper, and serve.

Blanched Dandelion Greens

Dandelions are considered to be weeds by most people, but they make delicious, sustainable salads.

SERVES 4

700–800g dandelion greens, *trimmed*
juice of 2 lemons
1 tablespoon organic butter
sea salt and freshly ground black pepper, to taste

1. Bring a large saucepan of salted water to the boil. Once boiling, reduce the heat and throw in the dandelions. Cook for 3–4 minutes, or until softened. Remove from the heat and drain.
2. Transfer to a serving dish, add the lemon juice and butter, season with salt and pepper, and toss.

You'll Never Eat Kale Another Way After This

Kale is a polarising food, and I totally get it. I've got recipes for fried kale, baked kale and sautéed kale, but this recipe is properly delish. This is a great veggie accompaniment to a meat meal.

SERVES 4

4 garlic cloves
1 whole curly kale, *stems removed, leaves roughly chopped*
200g mustard greens, *roughly chopped*
100g collard greens, *roughly chopped*
juice and grated zest of 1 lemon
sea salt and freshly ground black pepper, to taste
75ml macadamia oil or olive oil

1. Place the garlic cloves in a large stockpot or saucepan, add enough water to cover the greens, and bring to the boil.
2. Once boiled, reduce the heat to medium and throw in the kale, mustard greens and collard greens. Allow to simmer for 6–8 minutes, then drain well.
3. Transfer to a food processor, add the lemon juice and zest, and season with salt and pepper. Blitz for 20 seconds, then begin to add the macadamia oil until a rich purée forms.
4. Adjust seasonings and serve on individual plates or in a serving dish.

SAUCES, DIPS AND DRINKS

Rustic Salsa

Making a salsa often means using a blender or food processor to reduce all the ingredients to tiny particles. I quite like seeing the chunky bits of a salsa, so I simply chop my ingredients. You can choose either method.

MAKES 100 ML

¼ bunch of parsley, *leaves roughly chopped*
¼ bunch of mint, *leaves roughly chopped*
1 teaspoon capers, *roughly chopped*
3 tablespoons olive oil
1–2 tablespoons apple cider vinegar
1 long green chilli, *deseeded and finely chopped*
pinch of sea salt

1. Combine all the ingredients in a mixing bowl and toss well.
2. Adjust the seasoning and serve with fish, beef, chicken, lamb or eggs.

Tabouleh

It rarely gets any fresher than a tabouleh. Add some fatty fish, such as sardines, for a bigger meal.

SERVES 4

½ head of cauliflower, *cut into florets*
½ bunch of parsley, *roughly chopped*
¼ bunch of mint, *roughly chopped*
1 fennel bulb, *trimmed and finely diced*
small handful of okra pods, *thinly sliced*
1 large carrot, *shredded*
5 tomatoes, *chopped*
1 cucumber, *chopped*
1 red onion, *diced*
sea salt and freshly ground black pepper, to taste

DRESSING

120ml fresh lemon juice
240ml olive oil
2 garlic cloves, *crushed*
2 teaspoons ground sumac
1 teaspoon ground cumin

1. Combine the ingredients for the dressing in a small jar, cover and shake vigorously. Set aside.
2. Place all the ingredients for the tabouleh in a large bowl and gently toss. Add the dressing and toss again. Adjust seasonings and serve.

Pesto

MAKES 1 JAR

1 bunch of basil, *leaves picked*
¼ bunch of mint, *leaves picked*
½ garlic clove
60g raw macadamias
4 tablespoons olive oil or avocado oil (or more if needed)
juice of ½ lemon
sea salt and freshly ground black pepper, to taste

1. Throw all the ingredients in a blender or food processor. Blitz for 20–30 seconds, or until fully combined. Add more oil if required.
2. Store in a jar in the fridge for up to 2 weeks.

Cashew Cheese

This can be a great addition to a salad or a raw veggie dish, providing some richness and fat.

MAKES 250 G

200g raw cashews
60ml water
2 tablespoons lemon juice
1 teaspoon ground turmeric
1 garlic clove
¼ onion, *roughly chopped*
sea salt and freshly ground black pepper, to taste

1. Soak the cashews in water for at least 2 hours.
2. Drain the nuts and place in a blender or food processor along with 60ml of water, the lemon juice, turmeric, garlic and onion. Blitz for 20–30 seconds, or until fully combined. Season to taste with salt and pepper.
3. Store in an airtight container in the fridge for up to 2 weeks.

Coriander Mayo

MAKES ABOUT 400 G

2 organic egg yolks
2 teaspoons Dijon mustard
375ml macadamia oil
2 tablespoons lemon juice
⅓ bunch of coriander, *stalks finely chopped, leaves roughly chopped*
sea salt and freshly ground black pepper, to taste

1. In a large mixing bowl, whisk the egg yolks and mustard. Continue whisking while you slowly add the oil until a mayonnaise consistency is reached. Stir in the lemon juice and coriander, and season with salt and pepper.
2. Store in an airtight container in the fridge for up to 2 weeks.

Horseradish Mayo

MAKES **400** G

2 organic egg yolks
2 teaspoons Dijon mustard
375ml macadamia oil
2 tablespoons lemon juice
1 tablespoon grated horseradish
sea salt and freshly ground black pepper, to taste

1. In a large mixing bowl, whisk the egg yolks and mustard. Slowly add the oil until a mayonnaise consistency is reached (add more oil if necessary). Stir in the lemon juice and horseradish, and season with salt and pepper.
2. Store in an airtight container in the fridge for up to 2 weeks.

Coconut Mint Dressing

This very simple dressing can be used as an alternative to yoghurt.

MAKES 300 ML

1 x 400ml tin coconut cream, *chilled*
juice of ½ lemon
6 mint leaves, *roughly chopped*
sea salt and freshly ground black pepper, to taste

1. Remove the coconut tin from the fridge, open and remove the watery component.
2. Place the coconut cream in a large mixing bowl. Add the lemon juice and mint and whisk together. Season with salt and pepper to taste.

White Barbecue Sauce

This sauce pairs deliciously with roast pork or BBQ chicken.

MAKES 400G

300g Coriander Mayo (see recipe page 243, omit the coriander)
2 teaspoons Dijon mustard
1 long red chilli, *chopped*
½ teaspoon cayenne pepper
1 teaspoon honey
sea salt and freshly ground black pepper, to taste

1. In a mixing bowl, gently whisk all the ingredients together. Adjust seasonings if desired.
2. Transfer to an airtight container and keep in the fridge for up to 2 weeks.

Root Dip

This is a great way to use up any root veggies in the fridge or pantry that might be looking a little sad. There are no rules, really, about the types and ratios.

SERVES 4

1 large sweet potato, *chopped into large chunks*
1 onion, *quartered*
½ bulb of garlic, *cut laterally*
2 large carrots, *roughly chopped*
2 parsnips, *roughly chopped*
2–3 tablespoons olive oil
1 tablespoon chopped fresh rosemary
2 tablespoons tahini
1 teaspoon chilli flakes
1 teaspoon ground cumin
sea salt and freshly ground black pepper, to taste

1. Preheat your oven to 180°C.
2. Place the veggies on a baking tray, add the olive oil and rosemary, and season with salt and pepper. Mix well to coat the veggies.
3. Ensuring the garlic bulb is facing down in the tray, bake the vegetables until cooked through – about 50 minutes. Remove from the oven and allow to cool.
4. Remove the cloves from the garlic bulb and transfer to a food processor. Add the tahini, chilli flakes and cumin and blitz for 20–30 seconds. Add extra olive oil if necessary.
5. Season to taste with more salt and pepper, if desired. The dip can be stored in an airtight container in the fridge for up to 7 days.

The Only Dressing You Need

MAKES 200ML

1 organic egg
150ml olive oil
1 teaspoon seeded mustard
3 tablespoons apple cider vinegar
1 garlic clove, *crushed*
¼ bunch of parsley, *leaves picked*
¼ bunch of mint, *leaves picked*
sea salt and freshly ground black pepper, to taste

1. Throw all the ingredients in a blender and blitz until the dressing has emulsified. Season to taste with salt and pepper.
2. Store in a jar in the fridge for up to 2 weeks.

Herb Butter

MAKES 175G

150g organic butter
¼ bunch of parsley, *leaves chopped*
¼ bunch of dill, *chopped*
3 garlic cloves, *crushed*
1 tablespoon capers
1 long red chilli, *finely chopped*
juice and grated zest of 1 lemon
sea salt and freshly ground black pepper, to taste

1. Throw all the ingredients in a food processor and blitz until smooth. Adjust seasonings.
2. Transfer to an airtight container and store in the fridge for up to 4 weeks.

Hemp and Cacao Spread

This is crazy-easy to make and gives you a high-fat, nutrient-rich snack.

MAKES 1 LARGE JAR

130g raw macadamias
130g raw cashews
60g raw pecans
80g hemp seeds
2 heaped tablespoons raw cacao
1 tablespoon honey

1. Place all the ingredients in a food processor or blender. Blitz for 30 seconds, or until smooth.
2. Transfer to an airtight container and store in the fridge for up to 3 months.

Avocado and Lime Dressing

MAKES 1 JAR

1 ripe avocado
juice of 2 limes
¼ bunch of coriander, *leaves chopped*
1 garlic clove, *chopped*
1 tablespoon olive oil
4 tablespoons coconut cream
sea salt and freshly ground black pepper, to taste

1. Throw all the ingredients in a food processor and blitz for 30 seconds, or until smooth. If needed, add more lime juice, oil and coconut cream until the consistency is right, and adjust seasonings to taste.
2. Transfer to an airtight container and store in the fridge for up to 7 days.

Tahini Dressing with Capers

MAKES 150ML

2 tablespoons tahini
juice of 1 lemon
½ teaspoon ground cumin
1 garlic clove, *crushed*
1 tablespoon capers, *chopped*
sea salt and freshly ground black pepper, to taste

1. In a mixing bowl, whisk together the tahini and lemon juice. Add the cumin and mix again.
2. While constantly whisking, slowly add water until your dressing is of a consistently you like. Add the garlic and capers, and season with salt and pepper.
3. Transfer to an airtight container and store in the fridge for up to 4 weeks.

Reconditioned Coffee

A simple way to upgrade your coffee. If you have deadlines or are looking for creative inspiration, then one of these is the answer to your problems!

SERVES 1

1 long black coffee, hot
1 teaspoon collagen powder
1 tablespoon organic butter
1 tablespoon MCT oil

1. Place all the ingredients in a blender and blitz for 10 seconds.
2. Pour into a mug and serve.

The Green Stuff

SERVES 1

6–8 kale leaves
1–2 celery stalks
½ lemon, *peel removed*
½ cucumber
2cm knob of fresh ginger
1 pear
250ml water, coconut milk or nut milk
handful of ice
1 teaspoon honey (optional)

1. Place all the ingredients in a blender and blitz for 20 seconds, or until smooth.
2. Pour into a glass and serve.

Cricket Protein Smoothie

Gone are the days when the only protein powders were whey-based. Now we have options like hemp, pea, brown rice and – yes – crickets! It might sound radical, but cricket protein powder is available at online health food stores.

SERVES 1

1 tablespoon peanut butter
250ml coconut milk, or nut milk of your choice
2 tablespoons cricket protein powder
2 tablespoons cacao
1 tablespoon shredded coconut
handful of baby spinach leaves
1 teaspoon honey
handful of ice

1. Place all the ingredients in a blender and blitz for 20 seconds, or until smooth.
2. Pour into a glass and serve.

Crickets and Greens

SERVES 1

6–8 kale leaves, *chopped*

1–2 celery stalks, *chopped*

½ avocado

½ cucumber, *chopped*

1 apple, *cored and chopped*

handful of baby spinach leaves

2 tablespoons cricket protein powder

250ml water, coconut milk or nut milk

handful of ice

1 teaspoon honey (optional)

1. Place all the ingredients in a blender and blitz for 20 seconds, or until smooth.
2. Pour into a glass and serve.

Cricket and Reds

SERVES 1

200ml coconut milk or milk of choice

handful of frozen blackberries

2 tablespoons cricket protein powder

1 tablespoon cacao

2–3 tablespoons unsweetened coconut yoghurt

1 teaspoon cacao nibs

2–3 tablespoons walnuts

1 small beetroot, *chopped*

1 teaspoon honey

2–3 ice cubes

1. Place all the ingredients in a blender and blitz for 20 seconds, or
   until smooth.
2. Pour into a glass and serve.

Sprout Smoothie

Sprouts are a rich source of phytonutrients and help with cognitive function and cardiovascular health.

SERVES 1

½ ripe avocado
small handful of broccoli sprouts, or any sprout
1 tablespoon cashew butter
250ml coconut milk, or nut milk of your choice
2 tablespoons vanilla protein powder
juice of ½ lime
1 tablespoon MCT oil
1 teaspoon chia seeds
1 teaspoon honey (optional)
handful of ice

1. Place all the ingredients in a blender and blitz for 20 seconds, or until smooth.
2. Transfer to a glass and serve.

Frozen Breastmilk Pacifier

This simple and natural idea serves as a soothing aid for bubs who may be teething and a motor control aid for bubs around four months.

MAKES 4

Approx. 100ml breastmilk

1. Express the milk and transfer to a sterilised ice cube tray and place in the freezer for at least 2 hours, or until frozen.
2. When needed, pop out an ice cube of breastmilk into a mesh or silicone feeder. Never refreeze the milk, simply discard if not used.

Frozen Breastmilk Popsicle

This is a really simple idea for bubs over six months old who are taking solids, but they can easily be enjoyed by older members of the family ... if you're game, of course.

MAKES 4

200ml breastmilk
1 ripe mango (or fruit of your choice), *fleshed removed and puréed*

1. Combine the breastmilk and mango purée.
2. Pour into sterilised small popsicle containers and place in the freezer for at least 2 hours, or until frozen through.

Strawberry Smoothie with Breastmilk

I have just brought my second son into the world and, while watching my wife breastfeed him, it occurred to me that nothing is more natural than mother's milk. It's high in nutrients, organic and has no cost to the environment. It may sound peculiar but no more so than consuming the lactate of another mammalian species (cow, goat, etc). This recipe is aimed at the daring among you who have full consent from the lactating mum.

SERVES 1

50ml frozen breastmilk (2 ice cubes)
200ml coconut milk or nut milk of choice
handful of frozen strawberries
1 tablespoon peanut butter
2 tablespoons vanilla protein powder
1 teaspoon honey
handful of ice

1. Express the milk and transfer to a sterilised ice cube tray and place in the freezer for at least 2 hours, or until frozen.
2. Place all the ingredients in a blender and blitz for 20 seconds, or until smooth. Transfer to a glass and serve.

Endnotes

Introduction

1 Food and Agriculture Organization of the United Nations, 'The state of food security and nutrition in the world 2019', http://www.fao.org/state-of-food-security-nutrition/en/

CHAPTER ONE *From foraging to factory farming*

1 M Pirsaheb, M Limoee, F Namdari, R Khamutian, 'Organochlorine pesticides residue in breast milk: a systematic review', *Medical Journal of the Islamic Republic of Iran*, vol 29, 2015, https://www.ncbi.nlm.nih.gov/pubmed/26478886

2 P Nicolopoulou-Stamati et al, 'Chemical pesticides and human health: the urgent need for a new concept in agriculture', *Frontiers in Public Health*, vol 18(4), July 2016, https://www.ncbi.nlm.nih.gov/pmc/articles/PMC4947579/

3 R Wallace et al, 'Total suspended solids, nutrient and pesticide loads (2014–2015) for rivers that discharge to the Great Barrier Reef', Great Barrier Reef Catchment Loads Monitoring Program, Department of Science, Information Technology and Innovation, 2016, Brisbane.

4 FJ Kroon, P Thorburn, B Schaffelke, S Whitten, 'Towards protecting the Great Barrier Reef from land-based pollution', *Global Change Biology*, vol 22 (6), June 2016, https://www.ncbi.nlm.nih.gov/pubmed/26922913

5 Australian Bureau of Statistics, 'National Health Survey: First Results, 2014–15', December 2015, https://www.abs.gov.au/ausstats/abs@.nsf/Lookup/by%20Subject/4364.0.55.001~2014–15~Main%20Features~About%20the%20National%20Health%20Survey~3

6 EO Wilson, 'The diversity of life', Biodiversity Foundation, https://eowilsonfoundation.org/the-diversity-of-life/

7 Royal Society for the Protection of Birds, 'State of Nature 2013', https://ww2.rspb.org.uk/Images/stateofnature_tcm9–345839.pdf

8 Meat & Livestock Australia, 'Grazing strategies', https://www.mla.com.au/research-and-development/Grazing-pasture-management/native-pasture/grazing-management/grazing-strategies/#

9 I Tree, *Wilding*, Pan Macmillan Australia, Sydney, 2019.

CHAPTER TWO *Is eating animal products good for us . . . and the environment?*

1 A Simopoulos, 'An increase in the Omega-6/Omega-3 Fatty Acid Ratio increases the risk for obesity', *Nutrients*, vol 8(3), March 2016, https://www.ncbi.nlm.nih.gov/pmc/articles/PMC4808858/

2 Meat & Livestock Australia, 'Fast Facts 2018', https://www.mla.com.au/globalassets/mla-corporate/prices--markets/documents/trends--analysis/fast-facts--maps/mla_beef-fast-facts-2018.pdf

3 M Mellon, B Benbrook, K Lutz Benbrook, 'Hogging it: estimates of antimicrobial abuse in livestock', *Union of Concerned Scientists*, January 2001, https://www.ucsusa.org/food_and_agriculture/our-failing-food-system/industrial-agriculture/hogging-it-estimates-of.html

4 Food Safety & Sustainability Center, 'Beef Report', *Consumer Reports*, August 2015, https://advocacy.consumerreports.org/wp-content/uploads/2019/03/CR_FSASC_BeefReport_Aug2015-1-1.pdf

5   LA Horrocks, YK Yeo, 'Health benefits of docosahexaenoic acid (DHA)', *Pharmacol Res*, vol 40(3), September 1999, pp. 211–25, https://www.ncbi.nlm.nih.gov/pubmed/10479465

6   Greenpeace, 'Monsters of the oceans: 7 criminal super trawlers that threaten our waters', 19 November 2014, https://www.greenpeace.org.au/blog/monsters-oceans-7-criminal-super-trawlers-threaten-waters/

7   World Wildlife Fund, 'Overfishing: Overview', https://www.worldwildlife.org/threats/overfishing

8   The British Deer Society, 2015, https://www.bds.org.uk/index.php/advice-education/why-manage-deer

CHAPTER THREE   **Is veganism the answer?**

1   Z Harcombe, 'The EAT-Lancet diet is nutritionally deficient', 17 January 2019, https://www.zoeharcombe.com/2019/01/the-eat-lancet-diet-is-nutritionally-deficient/

2   G Ede, 'EAT-Lancet's plant-based planet: 10 things you need to know', January 2019, https://www.psychologytoday.com/us/blog/diagnosis-diet/201901/eat-lancets-plant-based-planet-10-things-you-need-know

3   C Kresser, 'RHR: What the EAT-*Lancet* paper gets wrong, with Diana Rodgers', 26 February 2019, https://chriskresser.com/what-the-eat-lancet-paper-gets-wrong-with-diana-rodgers/

4   R Moss, '3.5 million people in the UK are now vegan', *Huffington Post*, 4 April 2018, https://www.huffingtonpost.com.au/entry/35-million-people-in-the-uk-are-now-vegan_uk_5ac49b5ee4b093a1eb2087cb

5   M Archer, 'Ordering the vegetarian meal? There's more animal blood on your hands', *The Conversation*, 16 December 2011, https://theconversation.com/ordering-the-vegetarian-meal-theres-more-animal-blood-on-your-hands-4659

6   U.S. Food and Drug Administration, 'Foot Defect Levels Handbook', February 2005, www.fda.gov/food/ingredients-additives-gras-packaging-guidance-documents-regulatory-information/food-defect-levels-handbook#CHPTA

7   C Darwin, *The Power of Movement in Plants*, John Murray, London, 1880.

8   S Mancuso, 'The roots of plant intelligence', TedGlobal, July 2010, https://www.ted.com/talks/stefano_mancuso_the_roots_of_plant_intelligence

CHAPTER FOUR   **Is keto sustainable for you and the planet?**

1   C Kresser, 'Why your genes aren't your destiny', 24 February 2015, https://chriskresser.com/why-your-genes-arent-your-destiny/

2   C Choi, 'How epigenetics affects twins', *The Scientist*, 7 July 2005, https://www.the-scientist.com/research-round-up/how-epigenetics-affects-twins-48565

CHAPTER FIVE   **Daily rhythms**

1   Dr S Panda, *The Circadian Code*, Penguin Books, Sydney, 2018.

2   JD Plautz, M Kaneko, JC Hal, SA Kay, 'Independent photoreceptive circadian clocks throughout Drosophila', *Science*, vol 278, November 1997, https://www.ncbi.nlm.nih.gov/pubmed/9374465

3   Dr Satchin Panda, *The Circadian Code*, Penguin Books, Sydney, 2018.

4   Dr Satchin Panda, *The Circadian Code*, Penguin Books, Sydney, 2018.

5 ND Kohatsu et al, 'Sleep duration and body mass index in a rural population', *Archives of Internal Medicine*, vol 166(16), September 2006, https://www.ncbi.nlm.nih.gov/pubmed/16983047

6 EM Taveras et al, 'Short sleep duration in infancy and risk of childhood overweight', *Archives of Pediatrics & Adolescent Medicine*, 162(4), April 2008, p. 305, https://www.ncbi.nlm.nih.gov/pubmed/18391138

7 KL Knutson et al, 'Role of sleep duration and quality in the risk and severity of type 2 diabetes mellitus', *Archives of Internal Medicine*, 166(16), September 2006, p. 1768 *and* DJ Gottlieb et al, 'Association of sleep time with diabetes mellitus and impaired glucose tolerance', *Archives of Internal Medicine*, 165(8), April 2005, p. 863.

8 PM Nilsson et al, 'Incidence of diabetes in middle-aged men is related to sleep disturbances', *Diabetes Care*, 27(10), 2004, p. 2464.

9 CR King et al, 'Short sleep duration and incident coronary artery calcification', *Journal of the American Medical Association*, 300(24), December 2008, https://www.ncbi.nlm.nih.gov/pubmed/19109114

10 E Kasasbeh et al, 'Inflammatory aspects of sleep apnea and their cardiovascular consequences', *Southern Medical Journal*, 99(1), January 2006, p. 58–67, https://www.ncbi.nlm.nih.gov/pubmed/16466124

11 MR Opp et al. 'Neural-Immune interactions in the regulation of sleep', *Frontiers in Bioscience*, vol 8, May 2003, https://www.ncbi.nlm.nih.gov/pubmed/12700057

12 S Cohen et al. 'Sleep habits and susceptibility to the common cold', *Archives of Internal Medicine*, vol 169(1), January 2009, https://www.ncbi.nlm.nih.gov/pubmed/19139325

13 C Thaiss et al, 'Transkingdom control of microbiota diurnal oscillations promotes metabolic homeostasis', *Cell*, October 2014, http://www.cell.com/cell/retrieve/pii/S0092867414012367?_returnURL=https%3A%2F%2Flinkinghub.elsevier.com%2Fretrieve%2Fpii%2FS0092867414012367%3Fshowall%3Dtrue

14 J Bartholomew et al, 'Effects of acute exercise on mood and well-being in patients with major depressive disorder', *Medicine & Science in Sports and Exercise*, vol 37 (12), December 2005, https://journals.lww.com/acsm-msse/Fulltext/2005/12000/Effects_of_Acute_Exercise_on_Mood_and_Well_Being.3.aspx

CHAPTER SIX *Investing in your health*

1 Z Cormier, 'Did Neanderthals learn to make fire before us?', *BBC Earth*, https://www.bbcearth.com/blog/?article=did-neanderthals-learn-to-make-fire-before-homo-sapiens

2 D Sangathe, H Dibble, 'Who started the first fire?', *Sapiens*, 26 January 2017, https://www.sapiens.org/archaeology/neanderthal-fire/

3 J Adler, 'Why fire makes us human', *Smithsonian*, June 2013, https://www.smithsonianmag.com/science-nature/why-fire-makes-us-human-72989884/

4 Y Chen et al, 'High spicy food intake and risk of cancer: a meta-analysis of case–control studies', *Chinese Medical Journal*, vol 130(18), September 2017, https://www.researchgate.net/publication/319473368_High_Spicy_Food_Intake_and_Risk_of_Cancer_A_Meta-analysis_of_Case-control_Studies

5 M Chopan, B Littenberg, 'The association of hot red chili pepper consumption and mortality: a large population-based cohort study', *PLOS One*, vol 12(1), January 2017, https://www.ncbi.nlm.nih.gov/pmc/articles/PMC5222470/

6 S Freeman, 'How salt works', *How Stuff Works*, https://science.howstuffworks.com/innovation/edible-innovations/salt5.htm

7 National Health and Medical Research Council, 'Nutrient Reference Values for Australia and New Zealand: Sodium', September 2017, https://www.nrv.gov.au/nutrients/sodium

8 I Milne, 'Who was James Lind, and what exactly did he achieve', *The James Lind Library Bulletin*, https://www.jameslindlibrary.org/articles/who-was-james-lind-and-what-exactly-did-he-achieve/

9 R Ross, S Morgan, C Hill, 'Preservation and fermentation: past, present and future', *International Journal of Food Microbiology*, vol 79, November 2002, pp. 3–16.

CHAPTER SEVEN **Conclusion**

1 M Pollan, 'Power steer', *The New York Times Magazine*, 31 March 2002, https://www.nytimes.com/2002/03/31/magazine/power-steer.html

Further reading

Simon Fairlie, *Meat: A benign extravagance*, Permanent Publications, London, 2010.

Damon Gameau, *2040: A handbook for the regeneration*, Pan Macmillan Australia, Sydney, 2019.

Scott Gooding, *The Keto Diet: A 60-Day protocol to amplify your health*, Hachette Australia, Sydney, 2018.

Scott Gooding, *The Keto Diet Cookbook*, Hachette Australia, Sydney, 2018.

Dr Satchin Panda, *The Circadian Code: Lose weight, supercharge your energy and sleep well every night*, Penguin Books, Sydney, 2018.

Michael Pollan, *The Omnivore's Dilemma: A natural history of four meals*, Penguin Putnam, New York, 2007.

Isabella Tree, *Wilding: The return of nature to a British farm*, Pan Macmillan Australia, Sydney, 2019.

Matthew Walker, *Why We Sleep: The new science of sleep and dreams*, Penguin Books, London, 2018.

Acknowledgements

I'd first like to acknowledge my wonderfully witty, beautiful and effervescent wife, Matilda. Without her love and support I'd be blundering around in the dark. Thank you for bringing a lightness to my world, one which makes life a thousand times more fun.

I'd also like to acknowledge my in-laws, in particular my mother-in-law, Rachel, for not only contributing a delicious chicken recipe to the book but for being so damn passionate about animal welfare, regenerative farming and for fuelling those conversations.

A special nod to my mother and late father for imprinting such indelible impressions on me with regard to food, ingredients and flavours. After seeing how hard you both worked in your many pubs in and around London for close to 40 years, I swore hospitality would be a profession I'd never walk into, but lo and behold I've entered that world and feel all that much closer to you.

And a big thank you to all the farmers I had the pleasure to interview for this book, in particular Mick and Dom, as well as nutritionist Michelle Yandle.

Follow Scott online on
scottgoodingproject.com | reconditioned.me | thegoodplace.co

Facebook
Scott Gooding Project

Twitter
@scottgoodingpro

Instagram
@scottgoodingproject | @reconditioned.me

Index

agriculture
  animal deaths resulting from 51–2
  intensive xiv, 12, 16, 17, 27
  monocropping 12-13
AHR gene 109
algal oil 56
Alzheimer's disease 29, 53, 71
animal products, nutritional values 37
animals
  domestication 11
  ethical husbandry 7, 25–7, 34, 38, 124
  welfare 7, 33
Aquaculture Stewardship Council (ASC)
    41
Archer, Professor Mike 51, 52
autophagy 89, 90

beef
  antibiotics 27, 30, 32, 34
  feedlot-finished 20, 31–2, 33, 35
  grass-fed/-finished 30–1, 33–4
  growth hormones 31
  methane production ix, 25, 33
  rumen fistula 32–3
biomass 17–18, 19, 22, 65
body shape 73–4
Bolivia 125–6
Bourdain, Anthony 61, 62
Brain Derived Neurotrophic Factor
    (BDNF) 6, 71, 75, 97, 115

carbon 21, 25, 33, 65
carbon dioxide 33
cardiovascular function 84, 91
  sleep deficiency and 92
cattle see beef
cell grazing 21–2
cellular health 73, 102, 120
chicken 36–7
chilli 115
circadian rhythm 83–7
coeliac disease 6, 53
cold symptoms
  sleep deficiency and 92–3
cooking 107–9
  fish 111–12
  meat 110–12

'resting' meat 111
  vegetables 112–13
coral bleaching 15
cost of food 44–5

dams 22
dementia 53
desertification 24
  reversal 25
DHA nutrient 38
diabetes 16–7, 29
  sleep deficiency and 91–2
digestive system 87–90, 100, 102
diseases 16–17
  non-communicable 16
DIY growing/making 106–7

EAT-Lancet diet 48–50
ecosystems, diverse 12
Ede, Georgia 49
eggs 26, 55
Elinav, Professor Eran 93
epigenetics 8, 76–81, 97
  external influences 77
ethical animal husbandry 7, 25–7, 34, 38,
    124
exercise 6–7, 96–100
  incidental activities 98

farmers
  ethical 7, 25–7, 34, 38, 124
  role in climate change ix
farmers' markets 107
farming
  development 9–11
  family farms 11
  intensive xiv, 12, 16, 17, 27
  monocropping 12
  regenerative ix, 22, 27, 124
  underground 27–8
fasting 89–90
feedlots 20, 31–2, 35
fermented foods 118–19
fertilisers x, 14–15, 27, 66
fire 109
fish
  Aquaculture Stewardship Council
      (ASC) 41

fish (*continued*)
  cooking 111–12
  DHA nutrient 37–8
  farmed 40
  illegal practices 39
  Marine Stewardship Council (MSC)
    39, 41
  overfishing 38–9
food sovereignty 82, 125
frozen foods 106
Fubini, Dr Susan 32–3
fungi 17, 65–6

glomalin 65
gluten 6, 53–4
gluten-free diets 6
glycation 53–4
Grass Roots Urban Butchery (GRUB)
  25–7
Great Barrier Reef 15
Green, Mick x, 21–2, 44, 124
grow your own food 106–7
Gulf of Mexico 14–15
gut health 6, 18, 60, 119, 124

Harcombe, Zoë 48
health xv, 5, 8, 28, 44–5, 73
  cellular 73, 102, 120
heart disease x, 16, 92
herbivores 20
herbs 114–15
hunter–gatherers 9–10
  Hadza tribes 18, 34
hydroponically grown crops 18

immune function
  sleep deficiency and 92
Indigenous Australians 59, 114
inflammation 6, 53, 71, 89, 92
insects 55–6, 58–60
  farmed 60
insulin sensitivity 70–1, 88–9, 105
intensive farming xiv, 12, 16, 17, 27
iodine 116
iron 37, 54, 57, 118

jet-lag 93
junk food 79–81

keto diet 67
  'dirty keto' 72–3
  fat loss, encouragement 72
  foods, keto-friendly 75

health benefits 70
  inflammation reduction 71
  insulin sensitivity, improved 70–1,
    88–9
  ketosis, meaning 67
  mood and cognitive function 70
  neuron protection 71
Kresser, Chris 49, 77–8
  The Paleo Cure 49

lamb and mutton 34–5
  feedlots 35
  live sheep export 34
lemons 117–18
Lind, James 117, 118

Mancuso, Professor Stefano 64
Marine Stewardship Council (MSC)
  39, 41
meat *see also* beef; lamb and mutton
  anti-meat documentaries 43
  cheaper cuts 104
  consumption 7, 29
  cooking 110–12
  nutritional values 37
  offal 61
  'resting' meat 111
  synthetic lab-made 60–3
  whole animal purchases 104–5
melatonin 84, 85, 94
microbiome 18, 34, 60, 119
mitochondrial health 70, 73, 89, 120
'Move, Mob, Mow' 19–21, 34
mushrooms 65–6
mycelium 17, 64–6

nitrogen 14, 15, 66
nutrition
  tips for proper 52–6
  unbiased information 47

obesity 16, 29
  sleep deficiency and 91
oils, industrialised 6, 31, 53
omega-3 fatty acids 31
omega-6 fatty acids 6, 31, 53
oysters 55, 64

Panda, Dr Satchin 87, 88
People for the Ethical Treatment of
  Animals (PETA) 63
pesticides 13–14, 19, 66
phosphorous 14, 15, 66

pigeon 42
pigs 35–6
    free-range 36
plants, sentient 64–5
Plautz, Jeff 87
Pollan, Michael 124
population, global 58
probiotics 119
processed foods 5, 16, 105
protein powders 56

rabbit, 42
real foods 55, 101–2, 122
regenerative farming ix, 22, 27, 124
restaurant and café food 44
rewilding 23
rhythms, daily
    circadian 83–5
    time-restricted eating 88–90
    when to eat 86–8
Rosenbaum, Simon 98

Salatin, Joel ix, 19–21, 25
salt 115–17
Savory, Allan ix, 24–5
shopping tips 103–7
    bulk purchasing 105
    cheaper cuts 104–5
    whole animal purchases 104–5
sleep 83–5, 90–6
    cycles 95
    insufficient, health consequences 91–3
    sleep debt 94, 95–6
    strategies for good sleep 94
soil health x, 12–13, 21, 22
source of food, understanding 7
spices 114–15
sprouted grains 54

staple crops 10–11
    nutrient deficiencies 10, 16
State of Nature report 2013 18
strategies for sustainability success 3, 5–8
stress 79
sugar
    addictive nature 81
    industry 47–8
supplements 38, 56
sustainable, meaning 5
sustainable diet
    example of key foods 45

time-restricted eating 88–90
tobacco products 47
transglutaminase enzymes 54
Tree, Isabella ix, 23, 25
turmeric 115

underground farming 27–8
unprocessed food 5, 128

veganism
    growth in 50
    impact on animals 51–2
    tips for proper nutrition 52–6
    'white' 53–4
vegetables
    cooking 112–13
venison, 41–2, 52
vitamin B_{12} 37, 48, 55, 56, 75
vitamin C 54, 75, 117, 118

Ward, Rachel ix–xi, 212
Western diet 16–7, 72, 119
Wilson, E.O. 17

Yandle, Michelle 57–8, 74–5

RECIPES

asparagus, chargrilled with egg 151
avocado
    avocado and lime dressing 251
    crab and avo smash 184

bacon and broccoli frittata 136
barbecue sauce, white 246
beef
    beef cheeks 188

beef tartare 172
burger patties 201
mince and aubergine, midweek 210
pesto meatballs 202
steak with buttery mushrooms 215
surf and turf with horseradish mayo
    164
BLT with black pudding 135
Bolognese, venison 204

bowls
  Gooding smash 145
  green bowl with cashew cheese and
     coconut mint dressing 143
BRT 144
breakfast
  bacon and broccoli frittata 136
  BLT with black pudding 135
  BRT 144
  crab omelette 133
  fried egg omelette 138
  Gooding smash 145
  green bowl with cashew cheese and
     coconut mint dressing 143
  omega bowl 134
  pea and pancetta omelette 142
  pea and pesto omelette 140
  scrambled eggs with pesto 141
  shallots, tomatoes and eggs 139
breastmilk
  frozen pacifier 259
  frozen popsicle 260
  strawberry smoothie with breastmilk
     261
Brussels sprouts, roasted 232
burger patties 201

cashew cheese 242
cauliflower bruschetta 180
chicken
  butterflied herbed chook 168
  chicken and fennel soup 166
  chicken cacciatore 200
  DAS (delicious Asian salad) 174
  easy Moroccan chicken 216
  one-pot chicken 194
  Rachel's chicken soup with preserved
     lemon 212
  roast butterfly chicken with harissa
     211
  skewers 156
chopped salad 150
coconut mint dressing 245
cod
  cod curry 190
  crispy cod with sweet peas 170
coffee, reconditioned 253
coriander mayo 243
courgette, chargrilled salad 176
crab
  crab and avo smash 184
  omelette 133

crickets
  cricket protein smoothie 255
  crickets and greens 256
  crickets and reds 257
  pea soup with crickets 173
  spicy fried 228
cucumber and yoghurt 225
curries
  cod 190
  lamb and roasted squash 192
  salmon 198

dandelion greens, blanched 234
dinner
  barbecued rabbit 218
  beef cheeks 188
  burger patties 201
  chicken cacciatore 200
  cod curry 190
  confit salmon 209
  easy Moroccan chicken 216
  fish Provençale 206
  fish stew, fuss-free 221
  lamb and roasted squash curry 192
  lamb mince with squash and
     mushrooms 217
  liver and potatoes 195
  marinated pork 220
  mince and aubergine, midweek 210
  one-pot chicken 194
  pesto meatballs 202
  porchetta 222
  Rachel's chicken soup with preserved
     lemon 212
  roast butterfly chicken with harissa
     211
  roast venison 219
  sage and chicken livers 208
  salmon curry 198
  sausage hotpot 196
  slow-cooked lamb with anchovies 187
  slow-cooked roast pigeon 214
  steak with buttery mushrooms 215
  venison Bolognese 204
dip, root 247
dressings
  avocado and lime 251
  coconut mint 245
  tahini, with capers 252
  the only dressing you need 248

eggs
  bacon and broccoli frittata 136

chargrilled asparagus with egg 151
crab omelette 133
fried egg omelette 138
leftovers frittata 178
scrambled eggs with pesto 141
shallots, tomatoes and eggs 139

fish
cod curry 190
confit salmon 209
crispy cod with sweet peas 170
fish Provençale 206
fish stew, fuss-free 221
haddock in caper butter 177
Hilton Niçoise with roasted new
      potatoes 154
Mexican tuna with grapefruit, avocado
      and fennel 161
mouth-watering baked salmon 167
pan-fried hake with caper butter 158
frittata
bacon and broccoli 136
leftovers 178

Gooding smash 145
green bowl with cashew cheese and
      coconut mint dressing 143
greens
crickets and greens 256
green bowl with cashew cheese and
      coconut mint dressing 143
green stuff smoothie 254
pan-fried 231

hake, pan-fried with caper butter 158
haddock, in caper butter 177
hemp and cacao spread 250
herbs
herb butter 249
herbed oil 230
Hilton Niçoise with roasted new potatoes
      154
horseradish mayo 244

kale
the green stuff 254
you'll never eat kale another way after
      this 235
kebabs with coconut yoghurt 152
kelp noodles with pesto 160

lamb
kebabs with coconut yoghurt 152

lamb and roasted squash curry 192
lamb mince with squash and
      mushrooms 217
slow-cooked lamb with anchovies 187
spicy lamb larb 179
larb, spicy lamb 179
livers
liver and potatoes 195
sage and chicken livers 208
lobster, barbecued with herb butter 183
lunch
barbecued lobster with herb butter 183
barbecued venison 182
beef tartare 172
butterflied herbed chook 168
cauliflower bruschetta 180
chargrilled asparagus with egg 151
chargrilled courgette salad 176
chicken and fennel soup 166
chicken skewers 156
chopped salad 150
crab and avo smash 184
crispy cod with sweet peas 170
DAS (delicious Asian salad) 174
haddock in caper butter 177
Hilton Niçoise with roasted new
      potatoes 154
kebabs with coconut yoghurt 152
kelp noodles with pesto 160
leftovers frittata 178
Mexican tuna with grapefruit, avocado
      and fennel 161
mouth-watering baked salmon 167
pan-fried hake with caper butter 158
pea soup with crickets 173
prawn cocktail salad with coriander
      mayo 162
raw green salad 169
roasted butternut salad 159
spicy lamb larb 179
surf and turf with horseradish mayo 164
tomato salad 149

mayo
coriander 243
horseradish 244
Mexican tuna with grapefruit, avocado
      and fennel 161
Moroccan chicken, easy 216
mushrooms
lamb mince with squash and
      mushrooms 217
roasted buttered 229

sauteéd wild 233
steak with buttery mushrooms 215

omega bowl 134
omelettes
    crab 133
    fried egg 138
    pea and pancetta 142
    pea and pesto 140

peas
    pea and pancetta omelette 142
    pea and pesto omelette 140
    pea soup with crickets 173
pesto 241
    meatballs 202
    pea and pesto omelette 140
    scrambled eggs with pesto 141
pigeon, slow-cooked roast 214
porchetta 222
pork
    porchetta 222
potatoes
    crispy rosemary, with mayo 227
    liver and potatoes 195
prawns
    prawn cocktail salad with coriander
        mayo 162
    surf and turf with horseradish mayo
        164

rabbit, barbecued 218
raw green salad 169
root dip 247

sage and chicken livers 208
salads
    chargrilled courgette 176
    chopped 150
    DAS (delicious Asian salad) 174
    Hilton Niçoise with roasted new
        potatoes 154
    prawn cocktail, with coriander mayo
        162
    raw green 169
    roasted butternut 159
    tabouleh 240
    tomato 149
salmon

confit salmon 209
    curry 198
    mouth-watering baked salmon 167
salsa, rustic 239
sauce, white barbecue 246
sausage hotpot 196
shallots, tomatoes and eggs 139
skewers
    chicken 156
    kebabs with coconut yoghurt 152
smoothies
    crickets and greens 256
    crickets and reds 257
    cricket protein 255
    sprout 258
    strawberry smoothie with breastmilk
        261
    the green stuff 254
soups
    chicken and fennel 166
    pea, with crickets 173
    Rachel's chicken, with preserved
        lemon 212
sprout smoothie 258
squash
    delicious baked, with herbed oil 230
    lamb and roasted squash curry 192
    roasted butternut salad 159
steak with buttery mushrooms 215
strawberry smoothie with breastmilk 261

tabouleh 240
tahini dressing with capers 252
tomato salad 149
tuna
    Hilton Niçoise with roasted new
        potatoes 154
    Mexican tuna with grapefruit, avocado
        and fennel 161

veggies
    sauteéd veggies 226
    pan-fried greens 231
venison
    barbecued 182
    roast venison 219
    venison bolognese 204